EVERY BODY

EVERY BODY
A Nutritional Guide to Life

DEREK
LLEWELLYN-JONES

With illustrations by Benny Kandler

Oxford   New York   Toronto   Melbourne
OXFORD UNIVERSITY PRESS
1980

Oxford University Press, Walton Street, Oxford OX2 6DP

OXFORD   LONDON   GLASGOW
NEW YORK   TORONTO   MELBOURNE   WELLINGTON
KUALA LUMPUR   SINGAPORE   HONG KONG   TOKYO
DELHI   BOMBAY   CALCUTTA   MADRAS   KARACHI
NAIROBI   DAR ES SALAAM   CAPE TOWN

British Library Cataloguing in Publication Data
Llewellyn-Jones, Derek
  Every body.
  1. Nutrition
  I. Title
  641.1   TX353   79-42754

  ISBN 0-19-217691-9

Phototypset in V.I.P. Palatino by
Western Printing Services Ltd, Bristol
Printed in H.K. by New Kwok Hing Printing Press Co Ltd

Foreword

What you eat, how often you eat, and the substances added to the food you eat have a profound effect on your health. You may be surprised to know that in most industrialized nations many people are malnourished—that is, they eat the wrong foods in the wrong proportions. On the other hand, many people in the developing nations are undernourished—that is, they don't have enough to eat. They are also often malnourished.

Until people are aware of the ways in which the right foods promote good health and, conversely, the ways in which the wrong foods can lead to ill health, they are unlikely to change their eating habits.

That is what this book is about. It is a book about the way in which human beings eat and absorb foodstuffs and liquids. It describes how you use food substances for the production of the energy you need to keep alive, to maintain and repair body tissues, and ensure that your organs function properly so that you can continue to enjoy good health. It is a book about the nutritive value of foodstuffs, and the relationships between diet, health, and disease. It is critical of many modern dietary practices and of the way we encourage ill health by choosing foods with low or harmful nutritive qualities. It aims to make you, the reader, think about the foods you eat, and question whether your eating habits are sensible or healthy.

Contents

1

Fat people are fat because . . .

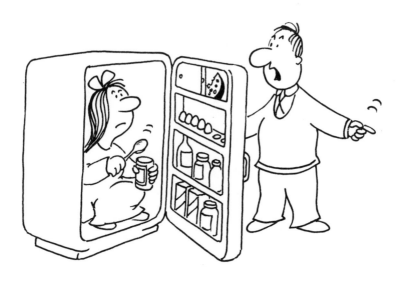

'If you treat cancer radically, either with surgery or radiation, you can give a person another three or four years of life. If you treat childhood obesity you can give a man another five years on his life span and a woman another eight years.'

Ciba Review, January 1973.

'Over-eating in an abundant culture requires neither courage, skill, learning, or guile. Gluttony demands less energy than lust, less effort than avarice.' *G. V. Mann, 1971.*

In Western affluent societies obesity is considered by many physicians to be a major health hazard. In this type of society most of us can afford, and obtain, a surfeit of rich food and drink: every day can be a feast day. Most of us can guard against heat loss by wearing warm clothes and by living in warm houses. Most of us need to take minimal exercise to complete our daily tasks. For these reasons most of us eat more food than we need, that is, we take in more energy (measured in calories) than we use. The extra energy is converted into fat and stored in our adipose (or fatty) tissues. As the amount of adipose tissue increases we become overweight. Some of us become obese.

The degree to which obesity is a health hazard is debatable. Dr George Mann, an American nutritionist, claims that only gross obesity carries health hazards. He is concerned that too many experts view obesity as a moral issue and write about it in a moralistic manner. The resultant guilt induced in fat people drives many of them into the hands of quacks—medically qualified and unqualified—or frauds and con-men. The quacks wax rich (and often fat!), while the obese victims, all too often, remain fat and guilty. Crazy diets, food fads, and dietary crazes cost the British public over £20 million and the American public over $700 million a year (according to Consumers' Association).

In poor, hungry societies, fatness is a sign of wealth and a protection against an unexpected famine. In our society, famine is unlikely and a protective layer of fat is unnecessary. However, according to the nutritionist Dr Mann, fatness has certain other uses—flotation, insulation, and flirtation. But since few of us spend all our time in water, and since most of us can insulate ourselves in cold weather with clothes and central heating, flirtation seems to be the only practical advantage of obesity! Unfortunately fatness is unfashionable in Western society. It should be stressed that this is a very recent cultural trend. Only since affluence has spread through our society in the past half-century has leanness been equated with beauty in women and with handsomeness in men. In earlier times to be fat was to be beautiful. Now health, youth, and beauty are inextricably associated with slimness. It is fashionable to be thin.

Dr Mann is correct in one way. The experience of many doctors who treat obesity is that the more obese someone is, the more difficult he finds it to keep to a weight-reducing diet. The decision to lose weight must, in general, be a personal choice, unless the obesity is so gross that it affects the heart or joints, or aggravates an existing disease, such as diabetes. In these cases the doctor may insist that an overweight patient loses weight. A difficult problem occurs when such a person refuses to take advice and appears unconcerned about the effects of gross obesity. But an even more difficult problem arises when a person who is only slightly overweight becomes unduly concerned and depressed.

Perhaps the best approach is this: if you are overweight and want to reduce your weight so that it lies within the normal range for your height, sex, physique, and age, and if you are prepared to accept the self-discipline of a slimming diet, then go ahead. But if you feel the ordeal is too great, just carry on eating.

Dr Mann's defence of moderate obesity is opposed by most physicians who have observed that obesity does seem to contribute to ill health. Obesity is frequently associated with diabetes, gall-bladder disease, high blood pressure, and arthritis. It may be involved, if only indirectly, in the high incidence of heart disease in Western societies. These facts, and the known higher mortality of fat people compared with people of normal weight, suggest that obesity *is* a major health problem in affluent nations. Furthermore, much of our obesity is due to our unwise dietary habits, which include our addiction to sugar and other 'refined cereals', and our over-indulgence in fats. We like our food too much, and we eat the wrong kinds of food.

It is true that from earliest infancy eating is a pleasurable experience, and when food is readily available we soon develop the habit of over-eating and may become overweight or even obese.

There are several ways of finding out if you are obese. One way is to weigh yourself and measure your height. Then you compare your weight on a chart made from studying the weights of large numbers of people of different heights (see opposite).

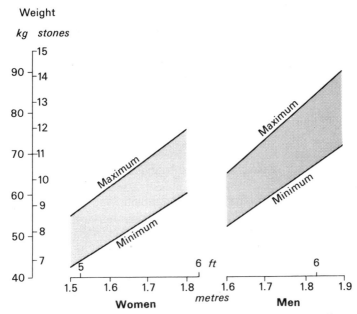

Maximum and minimum ideal weights for men and women of different heights, wearing indoor clothing

This method has the disadvantage that the measurement compares your weight with one which insurance company actuaries have determined is the most desirable to avoid disease and possible premature death.

Using the simple definition that an obese person is one whose weight is 20 per cent more than the ideal weight of a person of similar sex, age, and height, between 12 and 16 per cent of adult men and between 16 and 24 per cent of adult women in affluent nations are obese.

Important as that is, what you really want to know is how much fat you have in your body.

A simple way to find out is to grasp the skin and tissues over your lower rib-cage between your fingers and thumb. If the fold you pick up is thicker than one inch (2.5 cm), you are fat! This simple test for fat has recently been refined by scientists investigating obesity, or more accurately measuring the total adipose or fatty tissues in a person's body. They use special calipers to measure accurately the width of a fold of skin over the muscles on the back of your upper arm and a fold of skin below your shoulder blade. The first measurement gives a fairly accurate estimate of the fat stored on your limbs, and the second indicates how much fat is stored in your body, usually around your gut, and beneath your skin. Taken together the two measurements give a reasonable estimate of your total adipose (or fat-containing) tissues.

At this point a small problem arises. Adipose tissue is not made up entirely of fat, and adipose tissue is not the only place where energy is stored. Fat makes up about four-fifths of your adipose tissue (the balance being mostly water), but unfortunately the fat in the adipose tissues is only released slowly.

If you suddenly need energy, you obtain this from a second energy source called the 'glycogen–water pool' which is found in between your muscle fibres. You get energy very quickly from this source, but for each gram of glycogen you burn—which gives you 4 calories of energy—you also burn 3 grams of water.

If you are starving, which means little or no food and consequently no energy is getting into your body, at first you obtain the energy you need to keep alive from the glycogen–water pool (later you burn up your stored fat). During one week of starvation you need at least 6,000 calories to keep your body working. To get this amount of energy you will have to burn up 1,500 grams of glycogen from your store and consequently will also lose 3,500 grams of water. The weight of the glycogen and the water is about 5,000 grams, so you will lose about 5 kilograms of weight in that week. This rapid weight loss on a near-starvation diet is the basis of many quick weight-reducing diets, but they are effective only for a short period because the water you lose is replaced rapidly.

The only way to lose weight permanently is to lose it slowly by burning up your fat stores, and this takes time.

Applying the simple definition that an obese person is one who is 20 per cent above the average weight of people of similar sex, age, and height, about 12 per cent of adult American men and 16 per cent of adult American women are obese. In Britain, similar findings have been obtained. Both investigations show that in both sexes, but especially in women, the percentage of those who are obese rises with age, and there are more fat people in the lower social classes than in the upper classes.

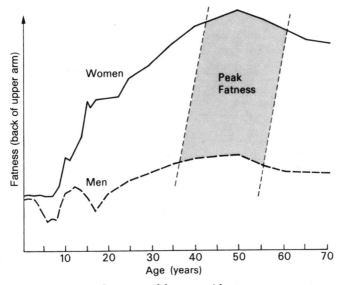

Increase of fatness with age

If obesity is so common, and if it carries a risk to your health, it is worth asking why fat people are fat. The simple answer is that fat people are fat because they eat too much, that is, they take in more energy than they use up. This is obviously not in itself a completely satisfactory answer, as many fat people claim, quite honestly, that they eat less than many lean people.

Most people have a friend who eats large quantities of food, who drinks a certain amount of alcohol, who loves sweets, and does not take much exercise—in fact who does everything which should make him fat—and who remains thin, or at least within normal weight limits. Such people discourage their fat friends who are on slimming diets. It seems so unfair!

Despite large gaps in our knowledge of why fat people are fat, scientists have sufficient information to make some reasonable guesses.

Your body needs energy to power the unconscious functions of breathing, heartbeat, heat control, and the other activities that keep you alive and which, together, make up your basal metabolic rate (or BMR). In addition, energy is necessary to replace worn-out tissues in your body with new tissue. Finally, every time you use your muscles consciously, energy is needed for muscular activity. All your energy needs are supplied in the form of food, and the energy balance of your body is calculated by measuring the energy absorbed from your food and subtracting from this the energy you expend in your BMR, in the creation of new tissue and in muscular activity.

Energy balance = intake–expenditure

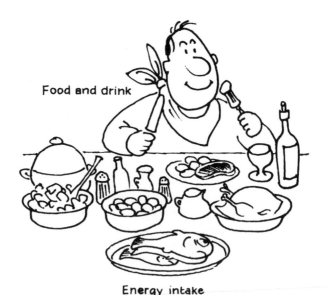

Food and drink

Energy intake

If your energy intake exceeds your energy expenditure, the extra energy is stored in the glycogen–water pool and in the adipose tissues of your body. The longer you continue to eat more energy than you use up, the more likely you are to become fat. So it is true to say that fat people eat too much while they are becoming fat, but once they are fat they may eat less than a lean person.

It is also probable that different people are differently 'tuned' to the amount of energy they use for their daily needs, just as cars of the same make and year may be able to travel different distances on the same amount of petrol. Some people approach a task in a relaxed manner and perform it with minimal extra activity; others use a good deal of energy in movements unconnected with the task, but which are important to their psychology. For example, one woman may cook a meal with economy of movement, while her neighbour flits about doing a variety of extraneous things when cooking the meal.

People whose bodies are finely 'tuned' to efficient energy expenditure may use up between 25 and 65 calories less each

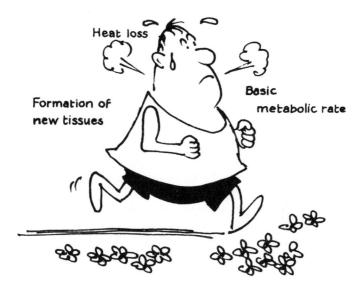

Energy expenditure

day compared with people who have a less efficient metabolism. If the two groups eat the same quantity of energy a day—say, 2,500 calories—a saving of 25 calories or 1 per cent of the intake, may seem unimportant. But over a period of ten years, 25 calories a day amounts to 91,000 calories. If this excess is all converted into stored fat, the person whose metabolism was more efficient would gain 13 kg in weight. On the same diet, doing the same tasks, the people with the more efficient metabolism would have become slowly, but perceptibly, fat.

There is some evidence, too, that fat people are less active than lean people. In a study using motion pictures of fat and thin girls playing tennis, volley-ball, and swimming, the obese girls were found to be inactive for twice as long as the thin girls. This lack of activity, which means in turn a reduction in energy expenditure, could be a factor in making some people fat.

Recently, another scientific observation has thrown some light on the problem. Most people know someone who is not especially active but who is able to eat as much food as he, or she, likes without ever putting on weight. For a long time there was no explanation of this, but scientists have now found that certain people are able in some way to increase their heat production, and then to dispose of the energy used to produce the heat by dissipating it into the surrounding environment so that, in fact, they use up more energy than expected. If it could be found what causes the increased heat production it might be possible to develop a drug which would make fat people become thin easily. No such drug exists at present.

It is possible that fat people lack this ability to dissipate heat and that there is an inherited, or genetic, cause for fatness. In other words you may be fat through no fault of your own but because you happen to have chosen fat parents! A study of over 40,000 children, adolescents, and adults in the U.S.A. lends some support to this view. The investigation was organized by the American Academy of Paediatrics. Doctors measured the fat fold in the back of the arm, which you may remember estimates the amount of fat stored on your limbs. They found that fat parents tended to have fat children, and that by the age of 17 the children of two fat parents were three times as fat as the children of two lean parents.

This would suggest that you inherit a tendency to fatness, but there is another, equally likely, explanation. This is that a fat person, whether a man or a woman, tends to choose another fat person as a marriage partner. It is likely that both have similar attitudes towards food: they enjoy eating and dislike exercising. They usually take large helpings of food and their enjoyment of food will be noticed and copied by their children. In fact, overeating probably starts in early childhood because fat parents equate a 'chubby' baby with a healthy baby and with good mothering. As you will see shortly, over-feeding in early childhood may be an important cause of adult obesity.

Fat families tend to have fat pets, which suggests that fat families overfeed themselves and their pets in the belief that 'fat is beautiful and healthy'.

There are other possible explanations for obesity. Most social entertainments provide food and drink which are additional to your normal energy needs, but the good company and the good food induce you to eat—in fact to over-eat. Psychological upsets play a part in over-eating, but do not appear to be major factors, as there is no evidence that obese people are more neurotic than thin people. Emotional stress makes a few people over-eat, others turn to alcohol, smoking, or drugs, especially tranquilliz-ers prescribed by doctors. Obese people who have emotional problems may have been conditioned in childhood to meet emotional stress by eating.

Most of us who live in the affluent world eat for social and psychological reasons as much as to satisfy the pangs of hunger.

An over-protective mother may condition her child by giving it sweets and other foods if the child is unhappy or hurts itself. A mother who says, 'Darling, I'll get you a sweet and you'll feel better!', at frequent intervals, may produce a fat child who later becomes a fat adult, because he has been conditioned to believe that food is an anxiety-reducer. When faced with stress or requiring solace, the conditioned person turns to food and becomes fat.

The variety of attractively packaged, precooked foods, espe-cially foods made of refined sugars and fats, such as sweets, canned drinks (including beer), cakes, and biscuits, that are available in abundance in shops and supermarkets may be a factor in the modern epidemic of obesity in affluent nations. The group of people who seem especially affected by the variety and availability of 'convenience' foods are usually sedentary, middle-aged women who belong to the lower social classes.

Many of these women claim that they are eating no more than they did when they were younger.

This may well be true. As you grow older your basal metabolic needs are reduced and you tend to become less active, so that you should eat less if you want to keep slim. As well as this, the middle-aged women we are discussing are likely to change the type of food they prefer. They may eat the same quantity of food, but in fact drink more cups of sweetened tea, eat more cakes and pastries, and enjoy more sweets and chocolates. These foods provide a high energy intake and make up an increasingly large proportion of the diet of many people.

Luckily, at least in youth when people are also more active, fashion plays a part in stopping many people from being excessively indulgent—at least, it deters many young women from gluttony. Fashion has today decreed that a young woman should be reasonably slim, and advertising, especially on television, has reinforced this view. This is understandable, since the current uniform of youth—tight-fitting jeans—looks ridiculous when stretched over fat bottoms and convex bellies.

To summarize, then, obesity occurs because, over a period of years, you eat more food than you require to meet your energy needs. But not everyone who over-eats gets fat. If you have chosen the right parents you may be lucky to have a metabolism which is 'tuned' so that you use more energy than others in doing identical tasks; or you may lose more energy, in the form of heat, than others who become fat. In addition psychological factors, to which you have been conditioned in childhood by your loving parents, and later by seductive advertising, may 'programme' you to need to over-eat. This last matter needs rather more consideration, as does the question of lack of exercise or sloth—to use an older word—as a cause of obesity.

Scientists both in London and in Paris have recently found evidence that the seeds of adult obesity may be planted very early in a child's life, and that misplaced mother-love may be an important factor both in childhood and in adult obesity.

The investigators examined the dietary history of fat babies. Since four out of every five fat babies becomes a fat adult, it seemed important to establish why the babies were fat. They found that most of them had been overfed from early infancy, and believe that this may be an important conditioning factor leading to childhood obesity and its usual sequel, adult obesity.

In recent years, over-enthusiastic mothers have been in the habit of giving young infants supplementary semi-solid cereals from a very early age. How this fashion started is not clear, but it has been encouraged by persuasive advertising and perhaps by the mother's desire for her baby to be chubbier, healthier, and better developed than her neighbours' babies. In our culture chubbiness implies good mother-care!

The strange habit of overfeeding infants with cereal supplements is a recent development and has coincided with the decline of breast-feeding. One hundred years ago most babies were breast-fed for the first year of life and semi-solid cereal supplements were only added towards the end of that period. Today, fewer than 20 per cent of mothers in many affluent nations breast-feed for more than two months. The 'formula feeds' are often incorrectly prepared, and mothers have been advised to add supplementary cereals to the formula feeds from as early as one month old, and certainly by three months old. These practices help the mother to obtain what she believes she should have—a chubby baby. Investigations in Britain and Canada suggest that over 40 per cent of babies are too fat. The overfat, chubby baby is produced by overfeeding, rather in the way a goose farmer stuffs his geese with food to produce *pâté de foie gras*.

What mothers have not realized, and their child health advisers have not explained, is that a mother may be doing her child a disservice by feeding it in this manner. Overfeeding the child in early infancy may 'programme', or condition the child to have a big appetite throughout its life. Such a 'programmed' child eats a larger amount of food before feeling full than an unprogrammed child. As a consequence, the child usually takes in more energy than it uses, the excess becomes fat, and fat children have an 80 per cent chance of becoming fat adults. By overfeeding her young infant a mother may be shortening its life, since fat adults tend to die earlier than thin adults.

In the last few years we have begun to understand why overfeeding in infancy produces fat adults. It appears that in the first year of life the fat cells in the baby's body increase in size.

From then on, overfeeding leads to an increase in the number of fat cells, which, once formed, remain permanently. This increase may occur because overfeeding fills the existing fat cells which, when they reach a certain size, split to make two cells and so on. It also appears that the more fat cells you have in the adipose (or fatty) tissues of your body the greater your need is to fill them. If a fat person, who was once a fat baby, tries to lose weight the cells simply decrease in size. The empty cells are thought, in some way, to stimulate the appetite so that dieting becomes difficult, if not impossible, particularly in a culture in which you are constantly importuned by advertising to buy processed rather than fresh foods. The potentially, or actually, obese child is likely to be given one of the sugar-coated breakfast cereals that now glutinously clutter the shelves of supermarkets, and cost at least twice as much as the original cereal from which they were derived, although they contain fewer nutrients. He is likely to buy sweets, chocolate, and ice-cream from the school tuck-shop, which is usually run by parents. His mother succumbs to the concerted efforts of high-pressure advertising to buy and try new, colourfully packaged, easily prepared, high-energy, 'refined' cereal products, and the child is likely to enjoy their sweetness, because he has demanding fat cells and is conditioned to a sweet taste. By the time he is an adult he is conditioned to want high-energy 'refined' food, and since his appetite is big, he eats and eats. And becomes an obese adult.

The conclusion of this research is that mothers who supplement their infant's feeds with semi-solid cereals from too early an age, and who give older children sweets, crisps, and peanuts as a reward for good behaviour are harming them, not helping them. They are being cruel, not kind.

Obesity can start because mothers in mistaken kindness overfeed their infants and children with foods to which sugar has been added.

Happily, this problem has diminished slightly in the last five years. An increasing number of mothers in the developed nations now choose to breast-feed; more mothers who bottle-feed use a modified (lower fat, lower sodium) milk formula than the full cream unmodified milk used previously by many; and fewer mothers are introducing solids so early in the baby's life. However, too many mothers still give their babies improperly mixed formula milk, and start solids too early. In 1978 a survey of 265 mothers in London showed that 47 (21 per cent) made the mixture 'incorrectly', and 164 (62 per cent) gave their baby solids regularly from the time it was 12 weeks old.

Of course, not all fat babies become fat children and then become fat adults. In fact about half the number of fat babies become fat children, and about four out of every five fat children become fat adults. However, only one in every three obese adults was fat when he or she was a child.

There appear to be two 'populations' of fat adults: those who were overfed as children and have more and larger fat cells than slim people, and those people who have persistently over-eaten, usually consuming a diet largely composed of 'refined carbohydrates' (sugar and white-flour products). These people have more fat in each fat cell, but do not necessarily have more fat cells than lean people of similar height. If the two populations of fat people diet, both will lose weight (provided they stick to the diet), but the obese adults who were also obese as children will find it harder to stick to their diet and even a slight period of food indulgence will result in a rapid weight gain.

As you grow older you need less food to meet your energy needs.

The pattern of over-eating over long periods accounts for most obesity, but not all. A few fat people have fat parents, and scientists believe that genetic reasons may account for their obesity. It is possible that certain women may lay down more fat cells during the development of the child in the uterus. This belief is still unproved.

Certain diseases cause obesity, but luckily they are rather rare. For example, some brain tumours induce obesity, presumably by affecting the hunger-controlling centre in the brain, and certain people who have rare endocrine disorders become excessively fat. But in general most fat people become fat because they eat too much, usually preferring foods that require no preparation, require little chewing, have a sweet taste, and are loaded with 'empty' calories.

Every body

Since it is so difficult to lose weight without great willpower, motivation, and persistence, it is preferable to avoid becoming overweight in the first place. Two of the seven deadly sins are gluttony and sloth. If you can avoid these two, you will not become fat and you may live longer to indulge in the remaining five—if you so wish!

Of course, if you enjoy gluttony and relish sloth, there is no reason why you should either diet or exercise. It is your life—but don't complain if your indulgence makes you unhealthy, uncomfortable, and perhaps even diseased.

Lack of exercise—sloth—is recognized as a factor leading to obesity. In modern society, automobiles, lifts, and labour-saving devices have diminished the need for exercise. Most people who take exercise now do so in a separate compartment of their lives, not as a natural part of everyday living.

Given a constant food intake, it is obvious that the more exercise you take the more energy you use and the less there is to be converted into stored fat. Unfortunately, you have to be very active to use up all the energy (calories) you obtain from your food. For example, a serving of breakfast cereal provides 100 calories; an apple or an orange, 60 calories; a 280 ml (10 oz) glass of beer, 115 calories; a can of Coca Cola, Pepsi Cola, or lemonade provides 150 calories; a slice of bread with butter and jam or a piece of cake provides 200 calories; and a hamburger provides between 350 and 500 calories, depending on size.

The amount of time you would have to spend on various activities to use up this energy is shown in the following table.

Energy provided by food in calories	Activity needed to burn up that energy in minutes			
	Sitting	Walking	Swimming	Bicycling
100	75	19	12	9
200	150	38	24	18
300	225	57	36	27
400	300	76	48	36
500	375	95	60	48

If you drink a glass of beer, you would have to sit for 85 minutes, walk for 21 minutes, swim for 14 minutes, bicycle for 10 minutes, or have a fairly torrid session of love-making to burn up the calories contained in the beer. This means that a good deal of exercise is needed to prevent you putting on that extra fat unless you also eat less, so that lack of exercise alone over the years is only a minor factor in your fatness. You become fat because you eat too much for too long a period.

However, using up extra calories by exercise can produce a significant weight loss, even if the amount is as small as 250 calories a day, as Dr Gwinup, who practises in California, has found. He studied 34 people who had failed to lose weight on diets, presumably because they failed to keep to their diets. He told them that they could eat their normal diet but they had to promise to take at least 30 minutes exercise each day for one year. Of the 34 people who participated in the experiment, only 11 lasted for the whole year. All were women! And all lost weight. The average weight loss was 10 kg (22 lb), ranging from 4.5 kg (10 lb) to 13.5 kg (30 lb). The amount of weight lost was related to the amount of exercise taken. Nobody lost any weight until she exercised for at least 30 minutes a day, and the 8 women who lost most weight exercised for more than 2 hours a day.

The participants chose whatever form of exercise they preferred and, not surprisingly, most chose walking rather than more vigorous exercise.

One hour's walking a day will use up between 250 and 300 calories; the same loss can be obtained by 35 minutes' bicycling or 25 minutes' swimming.

Exercise is therefore important in the treatment of obesity. It helps you to lose weight, and it improves your physical fitness, which is beneficial to you in other ways. It is also believed, especially by Dr Bjorntorp of Göteborg in Sweden, that regular exercise, especially after meals, may have a specific action in inducing weight loss, but unfortunately the effect is not constant.

There is a snag. Despite the current enthusiasm for jogging, most people are uninterested in exercise, or they appear to be, judging from surveys in Western nations. These show that four out of five people don't care about physical activity at all. Physical activity to keep fit and to maintain a lower weight is now not something we are interested in. Instead, most people tend to sit on their behinds watching television in their leisure hours, and avoiding as much exertion as possible during their working hours.

If the causes of obesity are many, the cure is apparently simple. Eat less than you need for the energy you use, exercise more, and your weight will fall. You will cease to be fat. Unfortunately, it isn't quite as simple as that, as you will see when you read the rest of this book.

It is often easier to make a desirable, if uncomfortable, change in habits if you understand the reason for making that change. Weight-reducing diets are all very well, but it is even better to understand the importance of good eating habits, so that the weight-reducing diet not only achieves a loss of weight but is nutritious and may effectively change some food habits which can lead to ill health.

To understand how bad food habits may affect your health and shorten your life, you may wish to learn more about the composition of your body and about the protein, the carbohydrates, the fats, the minerals, and the vitamins you eat. More information on this is contained in the Appendix.

The purpose of this book is to enable you to make an informed choice about the kinds of food and the quantity of food you eat. The choice is whether to go on eating unsuitable foods or whether to modify your eating habits so that you will lead a fuller, healthier life. The choice is yours.

People are conditioned by the foods they are given as an infant and as a child. Does the kind of milk you are given then make any difference to your future nutrition, health, and weight? The next chapter may help you decide.

2

Breast is best

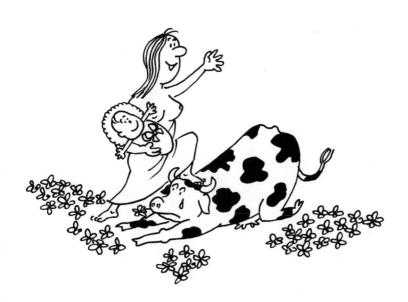

'In the present-day world's dietary patterns, the stress is increasingly on convenience foods, that is, processed foods that are precooked and ready to eat, possibly after initial warming. . . . Human milk represents the original ready-to-serve 24-hour convenience food, with advantages for both the father and the nursing mother.'   *Derrick and Patrice Jelliffe, 1971.*

From the evolutionary viewpoint the female breasts developed to provide the unprotected, relatively immobile, young animal with a means of obtaining food from a relatively mobile mother, until it ceased to be dependent on her. In humans, the dependent growing period has extended long beyond the period when breast milk is the young child's main food, but the principle remains: the mammary glands developed to provide food for young mammals.

In the evolutionary scheme of things, those activities that support life, or lead to the healthy development of an individual or a species, are associated with sensuous pleasure. For most of mankind's history, human breast milk has been vital for the survival of the race. It is small wonder, therefore, that the breasts are sources of sensuous pleasure. This pleasure is felt by men, women, and babies. Men find the shape of the female breast pleasurable and sensuous, either as a reminder of the warmth and security that their mother's breasts gave them as infants, or as a visible sign of female sexuality. Women know that their breasts give them a pleasurable sensuous feeling when stimulated by themselves, by a man, or by an infant suckling. A baby also apparently finds the breasts sensuous: an American paediatrician has observed that some babies, when sucking, make movements and sing 'nursing songs' similar to the spontaneous noises made by some adults during sexual intercourse.

Until about 70 years ago, breast milk and raw cow's milk were the only food available for infants. If the mother's milk failed, cow's milk was substituted, but this was a last resort, as it was correctly believed to be dangerous. Rich and fashionable women, particularly in the cities, tended to employ wet-nurses if breast-feeding interfered with their social pleasures, but at least the infant continued to receive human milk.

Since the 1920s technological advances in dairy farming and food processing, together with more stringent environmental health laws, have enabled manufacturers to produce processed, uncontaminated evaporated or powdered cow's milk. This made 'artificial' or 'formula' feeding practicable for infants in the industrialized nations.

The choice today is for a mother to breast-feed her baby if she possibly can—and over 95 per cent of mothers are able to breast-feed—or to feed him with modified cow's milk. There are important reasons why she should choose to breast-feed:

● Although cow's milk contains three times as much protein as human milk, most of this is casein. Casein coagulates into big curds which are less easily digested by the baby, so that the difference in the quantity of protein becomes insignificant.

● The quality of the protein in human milk is superior to that in cow's milk. Protein is made of 'building blocks' of amino-acids (see Appendix). Only two of the amino-acids contain sulphur, which is essential for growth. These are methionine and cystine. Before the body can make use of the sulphur-containing amino-acids, special enzymes are needed. These are normally found in the liver. The enzyme which enables methionine to be utilized is absent from the liver of most premature babies and some mature babies. These infants have to rely on cystine to provide the necessary sulphur-containing amino-acid. Human milk is unique in that it is relatively rich in cystine and poor in methionine. In contrast cow's milk, meat, and all other animal proteins have between 2 and 5 times as much methionine as cystine. Cow's milk therefore cannot compete with human milk in providing this amino-acid.

● Even more important, in view of the current belief that dietary fats may have some connection with coronary heart disease, is the fact that human milk has a high content of lineoleic acid compared with the amount in cow's milk. Lineoleic acid is a polyunsaturated fatty acid, and it is believed that polyunsaturated fatty acids are not likely to start the process of atherosclerosis, while saturated fatty acids may be a real cause. There appears to be a connection between bottle-feeding and the appearance of atherosclerosis in arteries. Dr Osborn, a pathologist when working in Derbyshire, performed autopsies on children and young adults who had died from various causes. He found out from their parents if the young people had been breast-fed or bottle-fed in infancy. When he correlated his two sets of findings he discovered that the adults who had been bottle-fed in infancy were three times more likely to have atherosclerotic areas in their aorta and coronary arteries than those who had been breast-fed for more than one month.

• Human milk contains an enzyme called lipase which helps fats break down into simpler substances. Cow's milk has no lipase. This means that the fats in human milk are partly digested before they get into the baby's gut, which enables the infant to absorb more fatty acids from human milk than it does from cow's milk. These give the infant extra energy, and provide the specialized lipids needed to clothe the connecting fibres in the human brain. Cow's milk contains the fatty acids but they are more readily available in human milk.

• Breast-fed babies, who are allowed to take as much milk as they wish, gain weight at an appropriate rate, because powerful self-regulatory controls in the infants prevent them from overfeeding. Cow's milk, on the other hand, particularly in the form of sweetened condensed milk, or dried milk to which sugar is added, tends to make babies overfeed, and may cause them to develop a taste for sugar. This may eventually cause them to become addicted to sugar, with undesirable consequences such as dental caries and diabetes. Early overfeeding of infants may also lay the seeds for the development, in later years, of diet-resistant obesity and possibly coronary heart disease.

• Human milk has a lower sodium and phosphate content than cow's milk, and most processed formula feeds based on cow's milk. The human baby's kidney has evolved over millions of years to cope with the sodium and phosphate content of breast milk. It was not designed to deal with the load found in many formula feeds which can be as much as four or five times that of breast milk. Unfortunately a few bottle-fed babies have kidneys which just cannot cope. These babies retain sodium and phosphate. The excess sodium makes the baby very thirsty and unhappy, and if the mother gives it another bottle the baby becomes worse. In some cases the excess sodium can even lead to brain damage. Retention of too much phosphate is not good for the baby either, as it may cause fits. These facts have led a team of scientists, commissioned by Britain's Department of Health and Social Security, to recommend that no baby should be fed on milk with a high sodium content, and if a mother can't or won't breast-feed her baby, a *modified* milk should be available in which both the sodium and phosphate content have been reduced to a safe level.

● Babies who are exclusively breast-fed for the first 4–6 months of their lives are seven times less likely to develop infantile eczema and gastro-intestinal upsets than bottle-fed or 'supplemented breast-fed' babies. These food allergies are particularly likely to occur if children of allergic parents are fed with 'formula feeds' based on cow's milk.

These are not the only advantages of human milk over cow's milk as the most suitable food for human infants. There is strong scientific evidence that breast-fed infants have a much smaller chance of developing infectious disease (especially infections of the gut leading to diarrhoea and vomiting) than babies fed on cow's milk. Some scientists, and many manufacturers of milk for 'artificial' feeding, argue that the increased risk for bottle-fed babies is caused by mothers who introduce the infection by making up the feeds unhygienically, but it is doubtful whether this is true in every case.

The advantages of breast milk compared with bottle milk are:
● **its quality is superior**
● **breast-fed babies are rarely overfed**
● **its fat content is more suitable for babies**
● **its sodium content is lower**
● **it protects the baby better against infections of the gut and pneumonia**

It is true, however, that even in developed nations formula baby feeds are often perfunctorily and negligently prepared and stored. In 1970 Dr Anderson and Dr Gatherer investigated the way in which English mothers sterilized bottles and teats they used for 'artificial' feeding. Health visitors visited 758 mothers chosen at random in large industrial towns, small industrial towns, country towns, and rural areas. They found that over one-third of the bottles, and nearly half the teats, were not properly sterilized, and that one baby in every five had been taken to a doctor at least once because of diarrhoea and vomiting. Mothers living in country districts were far more conscious of proper hygiene, and made more certain that the bottles and teats were not contaminated, than did mothers in the industrial towns of northern England. It is interesting, and worrying, to note that more babies under the age of one year die in the north of England than in the south.

Although contamination of bottles and teats by bacteria is a factor in the higher incidence of infection in bottle-fed babies, the evidence indicates that there is a *real* difference in the protective effects of human milk compared with cow's milk. In Scandinavia two well-documented investigations of babies born to women of reasonable intelligence, who were living in hygienic homes, showed that, in their first year of life, breast-fed babies had a lower incidence of acute diarrhoea, fevers, ear infections, and respiratory infections than bottle-fed babies. The bottle-fed babies not only developed more infections but these lasted longer and were more serious than those among breast-fed babies. In other words, breast milk seemed to give the infants some degree of protection against disease, especially gastro-intestinal disease.

The protective value of human milk is of even greater importance in areas where environmental sanitation is rudimentary or absent, and where there is much ignorance of personal hygiene and hygienic food preparation. These conditions exist to a greater or lesser degree in poor areas in all countries, but more particularly in the urban and peri-urban slums which are spreading in and around the congested decaying cities of the developing world.

In squalid, unsewered, largely insanitary slums, the pervasive and pernicious influence of commodity advertising, the need for many women to go out to work, and the decline in cultural peasant traditions have led to an increasing rejection of breast-feeding, with the disastrous result that large numbers of infants die unnecessarily from infectious diseases.

An example of the difference between breast-fed and bottle-fed babies in this situation has been highlighted by Dr Joe Wray, who has spent much of his life teaching child-care in developing nations. Dr Wray has observed that the effects of very early weaning or no breast-feeding are most severe in the early months of life. He found in rural Thailand, where most mothers breast-feed, that severe calorie–protein malnutrition is almost never seen in the first six months of life. In contrast, in some slum districts of Bangkok, where fewer mothers breast-feed, severe calorie–protein malnutrition affects as many as one baby in seven under six months of age. Dr Wray reports that children's deaths from certain infectious diseases were many times higher in Bangkok hospitals than in hospitals in provincial towns. He believes that severe calorie–protein malnutrition is the cause, and that breast-feeding prevents both the malnutrition and many of the deaths from diarrhoeal disease.

In China, where over 90 per cent of mothers breast-feed their babies, infant deaths from infectious disease are unusual. In fact the infant mortality rate (that is, the number of infants aged eleven months or less dying per 1,000 live births), is as low in China as in many of the affluent developed Western nations, and lower than in some.

Until recently the reason for the protective properties of breast milk were not known, but new scientific discoveries have begun to unravel the puzzle. In the first week of breast-feeding, the early milk, colostrum, transmits to the newly born baby protective antibodies called immuno-globulins. These substances are absorbed from the baby's gut and protect it against infection until it makes its own protective antibodies. After the first week or so of life, the baby seems unable to absorb the immuno-globulins from its gut, but breast milk continues to supply one particular immuno-globulin which stays in the gut and attacks dangerous bacteria and viruses if they should infect the infant's gut.

Human milk also contains other proteins, which are largely absent from cow's milk, and which protect the infant from gut infections. The two main agents are *alpha lactalbumin* and *lactoferrin*, which inhibit the growth of dangerous bacteria in the gut (particularly *E coli, staphlococci* and thrush) and prevent their absorption into the baby's body. Recently it has been found that human milk, as well as supplying protective antibodies and proteins, also contains large numbers of bacteria-killing cells. These cells, called macrophages, destroy two common gut bacteria (*E coli* and *staphlococci*) which often cause intestinal infections in babies.

The protective effect of human milk in preventing infections, demonstrated in the laboratory, is also shown in human communities. *Shigella* are unpleasant bacteria which cause severe gastro-enteritis. Scientists working in Egypt, in the Caribbean, and in Guatemala have shown that in countries where *Shigella* are common, breast-fed infants have few or no infections, but once they are weaned, or if they are bottle-fed, *Shigella* diarrhoea is common. In many tropical countries 'weaning diarrhoea' is a common cause of infant mortality.

It is also known that cow's milk, particularly if taken by infants less than two months old, may lead to allergic conditions, which often appear as unexplained 'tummy upsets'—either wind, or loose stools, or both. This is an additional reason for recommending breast-feeding.

Even if none of the advantages outlined so far tip the balance towards breast-feeding, there is one more significant reason for encouraging breast-feeding and for deploring its decline. This is the effect of breast-feeding on fertility and on the mother's health. Evidence derived from surveys in many nations suggests that breast-feeding tends to lengthen the interval between births. (The birth interval consists of the time from childbirth until the menstrual periods return; the time taken, once they have returned, for the woman to become pregnant; and finally the duration of the next pregnancy.) Lactation lengthens the birth interval mainly by increasing the time it takes for menstruation and ovulation to be established in many women. It is quite true that if a woman uses oral contraceptives or has an intrauterine device inserted, she will avoid pregnancy, but on a world-wide basis breast-feeding probably protects many more women from pregnancy (measured in woman-months per year) than are protected by conventional birth control methods. The decline in breast-feeding, particularly in urban slum areas in developing countries, has had the effect of increasing the birth-rate and adding to the grave problems of food shortages.

A lengthened birth interval is crucial for the health, the well-being, and often even the lives of women in the Third World. The shorter the birth interval, the greater the chance of mother or child or both dying. Ideally a woman needs between two and three years to recover completely from one pregnancy and to be properly ready for the next.

During this interval she may hope to replenish some of the nutrients she lost during pregnancy. If she becomes pregnant too soon, her body will still be markedly undernourished, and she will be at greater risk of producing a baby of low birth weight, and suffering from severe anaemia. The worse her nutrition after one pregnancy, the longer she needs to recover, and conversely, the sooner she becomes pregnant again, the greater the danger is to her and her unborn child. On average, a woman who breast-feeds will not menstruate for 8 to 12 months, and will be protected against pregnancy for most of this time. Conversely, a woman who chooses not to breast-feed will begin menstruating in 2–4 months, and is at risk of becoming pregnant again within two months, unless she uses contraceptives.

Until contraceptives are more generally used, breast-feeding will continue to be of great importance in reducing fertility, in improving the health of women, and for the survival of their children, in many parts of the world, particularly in rural areas and the urban slums of the developing countries.

Breast-feeding has other advantages over bottle-feeding, despite the seductive advertisements of formula milk manufacturers. Breast milk, is, as I quoted in the heading to this chapter, the original ready-to-serve 24-hour convenience food. The mother who breast-feeds has no anxieties about mixing and storing the formula feed. She need not worry whether she has enough supplies, if the bottles are really sterile, if the prepared milk is too hot or too cold, or if the teats are sterile or working properly. If she hears her baby crying hungrily, all she has to do is pick the baby up and give it her breast to suck. She is able to feed her baby anywhere at any time, provided that she does it discreetly. If she travels she does not have to boil water, prepare bottles, obtain foods, and go through the complex routine of preparing, feeding, and cleaning up. All she has to do is to let her baby nuzzle her nipple and guzzle her milk.

With the obvious benefits of human breast milk over formula cow's milk, it is difficult to understand why the proportion of babies breast-fed in the U.S.A. on discharge from hospital fell from 38 per cent to 18 per cent between 1946 and 1958. It is difficult to comprehend why in 1978 fewer than a third of mothers were still breast-feeding their children six weeks after birth in Australia, Britain, or Sweden.

Primitive races and groups invariably breast-feed their infants. Professor Ford investigated 46 preliterate groups and found that all the mothers breast-fed their babies. Admittedly one cultural group weaned their babies at six months and 13 at 18 months! But in 32 tribes breast-feeding was continued until the infants were two to three years old. In literate non-industrialized rural cultures, prolonged breast-feeding is also the rule. Dr Jelliffe observed that in rural Pakistan the majority of babies were breast-fed, at least partially, for about 18 months; and similar findings have been made in other Asian, African, and Latin American countries.

Until the 1920s the same applied to mothers in industrialized urban societies. For example, Dr Woodbury reported in 1925 that 58 per cent of 22,000 babies whose mothers lived in U.S. cities were still breast-fed at one year old.

In the 50 years between 1920 and 1970 the situation has changed dramatically. Today it is the exception to find a baby still breast-fed at six months old. Indeed, by three months of age, fewer than one-fifth of babies are still being breast-fed in the industrialized developed nations of the world.

In the past five years there has been a modest return to breast-feeding, especially among middle-class mothers in several developed nations. For example, in 1971 in Victoria, Australia, 20 per cent of the 75,000 babies born in that year were breast-fed at three months of age. By 1978, the number breast-fed at three months had risen to 40 per cent of the 59,000 babies born.

Despite this encouraging change, most mothers in developed parts of the world choose *not* to breast-feed their babies. The reasons for this are complex, variable, and ill-defined. One significant factor is the prevalent feeling in the West that nudity is indecent. The breasts are regarded as erotically stimulating, and this has engendered feelings of aversion to breast-feeding. Two English doctors examined the attitudes of 700 mothers to breast-feeding in the early 1960s. They reported that, 'for many mothers modesty and a feeling of distaste form a major factor in their preference for artificial methods'. At about the same time in the U.S.A. Dr Salber reported, after working among mothers who had refused to breast-feed, 'The idea of nursing repelled them. They were excessively embarrassed at the idea or too modest to nurse.'

As I wrote earlier in this chapter, the breast does have an erotic connotation, and the psychological responses of a woman to sexual stimulation and suckling are related. The womb contracts during suckling and at orgasm. Sexual stimulation causes the nipples to become fuller and erect, so does suckling. A few sexually excited women actually eject small amounts of fluid from their nipples. Breast stimulation by a partner arouses most women sexually, and leads to orgasm in a few. Suckling is a potent stimulatory trigger.

A woman who has been conditioned during childhood to fear sexual expression and to believe that the breasts are merely sexual symbols is likely to be emotionally disturbed at the thought of breast-feeding her baby. In turn, this negative attitude to breast-feeding is likely to make successful breast-feeding difficult and to turn the mother from breast-feeding to bottle-feeding.

Unfortunately, many attitudes learned in our society deter women from breast-feeding. The combination of childhood experiences in which talk and observation of sexuality is repressed and which elevates the breast to an erotic sexual symbol not a functional organ; and the experience at childbirth of impersonal, uncommunicative, authoritarian hospital staff are probably significant factors in the decline of breast-feeding in recent years. As well as this, the prevailing cultural pressure to have firm, shapely breasts causes some women to avoid breast-feeding in case their breasts become large or 'droop'.

There is very little accurate scientific information about the effects of breast-feeding on the subsequent shape of the breasts. In the U.S.A., Dr Oski tried to find out what the effect was. In a preliminary study he found that breast-feeding did not make the breasts permanently bigger, but the individual variation was as large as might be expected. Breast-feeding did cause an increase in the number of droopy breasts, but most of the women who breast-fed said that the pleasures of breast-feeding outweighed the slight tendency for them to have softer breasts.

A woman's ability to breast-feed successfully does not depend on the size of her breasts. Small breasts produce as much milk as big breasts.

A further factor which is causing a reduction in breast-feeding is that baby food manufacturers encourage bottle-feeding in devious and subtle ways. The baby milk and tinned infant food manufacturers not only advertise their products widely, but they also employ nurses to advise mothers. Much of the advertising and advice is excellent and encourages better health care and hygiene, but some of it is less than admirable. Women are subtly persuaded that the baby would do as well, or better, on the bottle, and it would be more convenient and less worrying to the mother.

This hidden persuasion is particularly sinister in societies where it is considered improper for a nursing mother to expose her breasts and feed her child in a public place, in which, for economic reasons, many women have to, or choose to, work. Few factories or offices outside Scandinavian and Communist nations provide facilities for infant care and breast-feeding. The belief of many child psychologists that mothers of infants and children under three years of age should devote their whole time to the child for the sake of psychosocial development may well be valid, but is ignored by the many women who choose to work (or have to work) outside the home, or who have social or sporting engagements which take them away. It is thought improper in Western society to take an infant to a lunch party and to feed it while talking with one's friends.

It is worth explaining briefly how breast milk is formed in the secreting areas of the breasts, and how it is subsequently 'let down' along the ducts and channels so that milk is available in the 'reservoirs' just below the nipples.

Dr Applebaum, who is the medical adviser to the La Leche League International, has described the breast as a 'forest consisting of 10–20 trees (lactiferous duct systems), all intimately bound together by interweaving vines and vegetation' (connective tissues, fatty tissue, blood vessels, and lymphatic vessels). These make up the structure and give shape to the female breast. In the innermost part of the 'milk trees'—in the clusters of leaves (the alveoli)—the milk is produced by specialized milk glands. The milk is squeezed out of the milk glands by a complex method, called the 'milk-ejection reflex'. It then passes down the narrow ducts which join the larger ducts to reach the main trunk ducts and to collect in the milk reservoirs which lie just beneath the nipples.

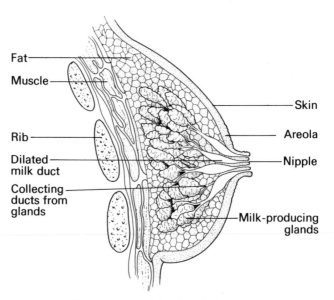

The structure of the female breast

During pregnancy, although the pituitary gland secretes the milk-producing hormone prolactin in increasing amounts, lactation is prevented. This is because the circulating sex hormones (oestrogen and progesterone), which are preparing the breast tissues for milk production, prevent prolactin from stimulating the milk-producing cells in the alveoli.

Following childbirth, the levels of the sex hormones fall precipitously and prolactin begins to act on the milk-producing cells. Milk begins to be secreted by the cells and to be released into the milk ducts. Prolactin is released into the blood-stream. It initiates and then maintains the manufacture of milk in the alveoli deep in the breasts.

At first, only thick colostrum is secreted, but by 24–48 hours after birth, milk appears and the amount secreted is regulated by the baby's demand. The process is helped if the mother wants to feed, and if the baby remains with her so that it can be nursed as soon and as often as it wishes, both during the day and at night.

The secretion of milk continues because prolactin continues to be released as the nipple is nuzzled by the baby or when the mother cuddles her baby. However, the secreted milk will remain in the milk glands, distending them, unless the milk-ejection reflex occurs. The reflex forces the milk out of the milk glands to run along the ducts towards the milk reservoir. This 'let-down' of milk is due to contractions of minute muscles which surround the milk glands. The muscles are activated in a complex way, the main component of which is the stimulation of the mother's nipple by a nuzzling baby. A message travels from the stimulated nipple along nerve pathways to the brain, and from there to the pituitary gland. The message tells the pituitary gland to release a muscle-contracting substance called oxytocin into the blood-stream. This is carried in the blood to the tiny muscles around the milk glands with the result that the muscles contract and the milk is forced along the milk ducts.

Milk-ejection, or 'let-down' has occurred, and is associated with a gentle tingling in the breasts and a desire to nurse. The reflex can also be initiated without actual stimulation of the nipples. A mother hearing the baby cry, for example, may feel the signs of milk-ejection. But the most potent stimulus to milk-ejection is stimulation of the mother's nipples.

Every body

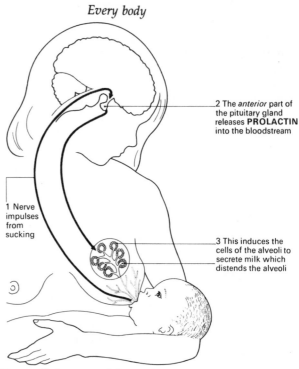

2 The *anterior* part of the pituitary gland releases **PROLACTIN** into the bloodstream

1 Nerve impulses from sucking

3 This induces the cells of the alveoli to secrete milk which distends the alveoli

How milk is secreted during breast-feeding

If the milk-ejection reflex does not occur regularly and adequately, the secreted milk distends the milk glands and the resulting pressure prevents further milk being made. The breasts become painful. If a mother says she has 'insufficient milk' it generally means that the milk-ejection reflex is not working properly, although her milk production is normal.

As the pathway of the reflex goes through the brain, the release of the oxytocin needed to cause milk-ejection can be affected by the emotions and by other psychological factors. Dr Niles Newton, a psychologist, and her husband, Dr Michael Newton, an obstetrician, talked with 91 mothers, and asked questions to which the women replied in writing. When the answers were analysed, Dr Newton found that those women who subconsciously, or consciously, showed that they disliked the idea of breast-feeding produced less milk. After a number of days this inevitably led to a hungry, crying baby, to greater maternal anxiety, and to the decision to 'put the baby on the

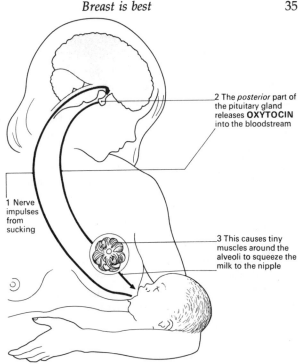

2 The *posterior* part of the pituitary gland releases **OXYTOCIN** into the bloodstream

1 Nerve impulses from sucking

3 This causes tiny muscles around the alveoli to squeeze the milk to the nipple

How milk is 'let-down' during breast-feeding

bottle because I haven't enough milk and it doesn't agree with the baby'.

The converse was also true. If a woman really wanted to breast-feed she was far more likely to succeed.

The Newtons found that fear of pain, a mother's anxiety about her ability to breast-feed, disparaging remarks about breast-feeding by friends, and an authoritarian, brusque attitude by nursing staff hindered the milk-ejection reflex and made successful breast-feeding less likely to occur. Dr Applebaum commented, 'A kind sympathetic approach by the nursing staff is important to over-all success in breast-feeding. Too many nurses hand the infant to the mother expecting her to know what to do.'

In many surveys in which mothers were asked why they stopped breast-feeding, the most usual answer was 'insufficient milk' or 'the nurse said the milk doesn't agree with my baby'.

To a large extent the mother's anxiety about successful

breast-feeding is aggravated by the practice, in many hospitals, of separating the mother from her baby. In many institutions the baby lives for most of the time in a nursery and is only brought to its mother at intervals for feeding. As babies are imitative, there is generally a good deal of crying in the nursery, and this is interpreted as hunger crying by the nursery attendants. To quell the noise and treat the supposed hunger, glucose drinks are given. The wide-holed teats and the sweet drink give the baby an easy feed, and it is rapidly conditioned to sweetness, so that it resists and resents having to obtain the less sweet breast milk. The partly satiated child, when taken at the 'correct' time interval (chosen by the nursing staff, not the baby) to its mother, is not interested in suckling. This in turn reduces lactation, because the reflex invoked by stimulating the nipple which causes prolactin release is reduced.

Breast-feeding is encouraged by mother and baby sharing the same room in hospitals, by helpful, motivated nurses, and by a reduction of hospital routine.

Babies fed 'on demand' gain weight more quickly (after the normal initial weight loss) than babies fed 'by the clock'.

Only when the mother and baby live together and are treated by unhurried kindly nurses, and when demand feeding is practised, will the emotional bonds between the two become firm. But all too often hospitals seem to be run for the benefit of the staff rather than for the benefit of the mother and her baby. This in itself is hardly conducive to successful breast-feeding.

The importance of this infant–mother bonding is that the tactile sensations stimulate the baby's sucking reflex and the mother's milk-ejection reflex. The more the milk-ejection reflex is stimulated in the first four days of life, the more successful lactation is likely to be. This in turn suggests that the reflex is started by more than the actual stimulation of the nipples. The close mother–child contact common in developing countries, and lost in recent years in our industrialized, mechanized societies, is a further potent stimulus to successful breast-feeding. The practices of allowing the mother and baby to share a room and of 'demand feeding' are a return to a more sensible and humane attitude and to a greater chance that breast-feeding will occur and persist. But unless hospitals encourage this return, breast-feeding will continue to decline.

Hospitals should abandon the following practices, as they discourage mothers from breast-feeding:

● Preventing the mother and baby having skin-to-skin contact immediately after birth, and initiating breast-feeding during this time. An active baby will seek for the nipple and suck within minutes of birth. It should be allowed to do so, as this initiates the release of prolactin by the mother, and enables the baby to practise its sucking reflex.

● Separating mother and baby during the first days of its life, and insisting that the mother only feeds at 3-hour or 4-hour intervals. If the mother and baby are together and the mother cuddles and feeds the baby when it cries, the experience will lead to a closer 'bonding' and to a greater, more persistent release of prolactin.

● Giving the baby glucose water before its first feed; weighing the baby before and after feeds and giving extra glucose water if the weight gain is thought to be insufficient. A healthy newborn baby has all the additional fluid it needs in its own body, and requires no extra fluids in the first days of life, before its mother's milk 'comes in' 2–4 days after childbirth.

● Separating the mother and baby at night, so that the mother sleeps all night and the baby is given glucose in the nursery. The milk supply will be increased if mother and baby sleep in the same room all the time and she feeds it whenever it demands milk.

● Preventing demand feeding. The baby should be fed whenever *it* wants food, even though this may mean 10 or more feeds in each 24-hour period.

● Offering the baby water sweetened with glucose after it has fed. Demand-fed babies rarely need extra water, but if offered it will usually take a small amount.

• Instructing the mother to feed by the clock at intervals of no less than three hours when she goes home.

These practices not only lead to breast engorgement and pain in the first days after childbirth (by hindering the milk-ejection reflex) but suggest to a mother that breast-feeding is a very complicated matter. This leads to anxiety and a feeling of inadequacy. The mother feels that she does not know how to cope with a normal function, and that she will fail to feed her child. This psychological upset aggravates the failure of her milk to 'let down' with resulting lack of milk for the baby.

When she goes home her anxiety often increases. She now has to cope with her new baby on her own and the baby seems to be increasingly fretful. She wonders if her baby's unhappiness is due to her inability to look after it properly, or perhaps if its fretfulness is due to hunger because her milk is not good enough or there isn't enough of it. So she rings up a friend or a neighbour or a nurse and is usually told that she should complement the breast milk with an infant formula milk or with semi-solids. This advice is the worst she can get—that is, if she wants to breast-feed.

It is important for nursing mothers to know the essential physiological principle of breast-feeding: the stimulus of sucking creates more milk. A breast-fed baby who is fretful and cries most of the time is most likely hungry. It needs to be cuddled and to be fed and the most logical way of relieving its hunger is to suckle it.

To succeed in breast-feeding a mother needs information and confidence. Organizations like the National Childbirth Trust in the U.K., the La Leche League in the U.S.A., or the Nursing Mothers' Association in Australia, all have counsellors who can supplement the advice given to mothers while they are in hospital.

Breast-feeding is not instinctive. It has to be learned. The best way to start is for the mother to be given her baby to cuddle and put to her breast immediately it is born.

Lactating mothers often ask how long they should continue to breast-feed without giving the baby one of the supplementary baby foods so persuasively advertised by the manufacturers. If a woman does not give her baby the appropriate sieved, mushed tin of vegetables or liver or meat is she depriving her baby of essential nutriment?

The evidence is that breast milk will provide all the nutrition required for a human infant for the first four to six months of life. Until saliva begins to be secreted at about 4 months old, and until the first teeth have appeared and a child has learned to chew, breast milk is all that is needed. These changes occur at about six months of age. At this time cereal, egg yolk, or banana can be started and the child can begin to eat 'off the table' without the need for expensive, commercially prepared, strained, 'convenience' baby foods. At this age too, a baby will start drinking from a cup, so that in many cases the bottle is not required at any time. The mother should begin to give her baby a variety of solids, and to establish proper eating habits. In the developed nations she is likely to buy tinned baby foods (although many of these contain rather too much salt and some have added sugar), or, more cheaply, she can prepare her own. In the developing nations, local cereal-legume mixes are more appropriate and considerably less expensive than imported baby foods. The mother may also continue to breast-feed (or bottle-feed), and partial breast-feeding can continue for a year or more if the mother wishes. If women did this the problems of 'weaning diarrhoea' in tropical countries, and those of obesity and possibly high blood pressure in developed nations would be considerably reduced.

The bias in favour of breast-feeding and breast milk for infants should not obscure the fact that cow's milk, whether raw or processed, or converted into cheese, is an important source of protein for older children and for adults, particularly pregnant women. If nearly all of the world's babies were breast-fed, a large amount of milk and milk products could be made available to reduce the present protein malnutrition which affects so many children in the developing world. Or, to look at it another way, if all the babies in Asia were bottle-fed an extra herd of 114 million cows would be needed. As it is, bottle-feeding costs at least $300 million a year.

It is also fair to say that if a woman cannot or chooses not to breast-feed, modern 'artificial' milks are adequate substitutes for breast milk, provided they are properly and intelligently prepared, and the mixing vessels, the bottle, and the teats are properly sterilized. Unfortunately, all too often, as I have mentioned, 'artificial' milks are not properly prepared under sterile conditions. Women whose babies are bottle-fed tend to be susceptible to a large amount of conflicting information about infant feeding. This comes from a variety of sources, such as health visitors, child health clinics, nurse employees of baby food manufacturers, general practitioners, paediatricians, relatives, friends, and child-care books. In some cases the advice is based on sound infant-care practice, but often it is based on habit or folklore. Often the advice is contradictory so that the mother becomes confused and anxious, particularly when her baby cries a good deal and appears not to be thriving.

In an attempt to find out the effect of this conflicting advice on the well-being of the artificially fed babies, Dr Oates, when a paediatrician at St Mary's Hospital, London, interviewed one hundred mothers of infants under six months of age and followed them up over a period of time. The results of his survey are disturbing. Forty-two per cent of the mothers changed to a different milk preparation in the period studied, and 26 per cent changed in the first two weeks after the baby was born. Nine per cent of the babies were changed several times. The reasons for making the change varied from 'no definite reason' to 'advice from the local chemist'. It is interesting that most paediatricians believe that there is little difference between the various dried milk products available, as far as the growth and well-being of the infant is concerned, provided the milk is properly prepared. Dr Oates found that no fewer than 59 per cent of the mothers were not preparing the milk as recommended by the manufacturers. One mother in every five made a more concentrated mixture than recommended, and one in ten made a more dilute mixture. The danger of making the mixture more concentrated than recommended is that the milk may have too much salt in it.

Although most babies can probably cope with the extra load, they are less able to do this if the mother has made a more concentrated mixture than the directions suggested. An infant fed on such a mixture may get high levels of sodium in its blood.

This in turn could lead to possible brain damage, as I mentioned earlier. It also makes the infant thirsty, so that it cries. The mother interprets this as an indication that the baby is hungry and gives it more of the concentrated milk. This leads to more thirst and to the offer of more milk. The extra calories from the extra milk may lead to obesity, and obesity in infancy is a cause of obesity in later life, as I discussed in Chapter 1.

The mothers of the artificially fed babies studied by Dr Oates also started giving their babies solids, usually, cereals, rusks, or tinned baby foods, early in life. Twenty-eight per cent of the babies were given solids (usually added to the milk) by the age of four weeks, and by eight weeks 55 per cent were getting extra solids. Not only is the early introduction of solids unnecessary, but the habit aggravates the likelihood of infant obesity and its consequences. Dr Oates commented, 'as infant feeding practices are largely influenced by tradition, folklore, and advertising pressures, considerable educational effort may be needed to avert the trend to obesity and the dangers of hypernatraemia (high blood levels of salt) to which many infants seem to be exposed'.

The dangers would be avoided, of course, if women chose to breast-feed. The reassurance to a mother who cannot breast-feed that 'artificial feeding' will not materially hinder her child's growth and development, provided the milk is properly and intelligently prepared, must be allied to a plea that, for most infants, 'breast is best'; and for mankind as a whole, the reversion to breast-feeding would have far-reaching desirable consequences.

Since the evidence is that formula-milk ('artificial') feeding is chosen in preference to breast-feeding because of embarrassment, because of a fear that the infant will receive insufficient milk, and because of custom, the steps which would lead to a return to breast-feeding should start early and should include:

● Education about human nutrition in schools. Both boys and girls should learn about the importance of breast-feeding and to perceive the female breast as an organ of infant nutrition as well as being a female sexual symbol.

● The education should be reinforced in early pregnancy by the medical attendants.

● After childbirth, nurses and doctors should encourage demand feeding and permit the mother to have her baby beside her for most or all of the time.

● Once the lactating mother leaves hospital and goes home she should be able to call for encouragement, counselling, help, and support from organizations and informed people.

● Allowances should be paid to extend the period of maternity leave for those women who breast-feed.

● For women who wish to work, or have to work, managements (and Trade Unions) should modify the working day so that breast-feeding can continue, and should provide facilities at work for breast-feeding.

Composition of human milk and cow's milk

Biochemical substance	Human milk	Cow's milk
Water per 100 ml	87.1	87.3
Total solids		
Protein g/100 ml	0.9	3.3
Casein % of total	20	82
Whey % of total	80	18
Fat g/100 ml	4.5	3.7
Milk sugar (lactose)	6.8	4.8
Minerals mg/100 ml		
Calcium mg	34	125
Phosphorus mg	14	96
Sodium mmol/litre	7	25
Vitamins per 100 ml		
vitamin A i.u.	190	100
vitamin B_1 i.u.	16	44
vitamin B_2 i.u.	36	175
vitamin B i.u.	150	950
vitamin C mg	4.3	1.1
Inhibitors of Bacteria		
Secretory Immunoglobulin A	+ +	Absent
Alpha lactalbumin	+ +	+
Lactoferrin	+ +	Absent
Lysofyme	+	Absent
Mother's macrophages	+ +	Absent
Energy Provided (kcal/gm)	**75**	**69**

3

Our daily bread

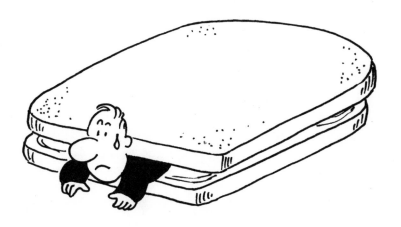

'The Lion and the Unicorn
Were fighting for the crown,
The Lion and the Unicorn
Fought all over town.
Some gave them white bread,
And some gave them brown,
Some gave them plum cake,
And drummed them out of town.'

Nursery rhyme.

'If I am hungry . . . I don't care whether the bread is black, brown, or white. My stomach wants to be filled, not entertained. *Seneca.*

About 40,000 years ago nomadic man learned how to make fire, and 30,000 years later he learnt how to cultivate grasses, whose seeds he had previously only picked. By judicious selection or, more likely, by trial and error, he began the conscious cultivation of barley and wheat. He gathered the barley seeds, pounded them, and made porridge of the result by cooking the pounded cereals. This astonishing advance in food technology was first practised in the foothills of the Tigris-Euphrates valley in Asia Minor, and spread as the nomadic tribes moved further and further afield. But porridge was relatively unsatisfying. It had to be eaten when it was cooked, and it was difficult to carry. By 2000 B.C. flat unleavened cakes of flour were replacing the porridge, and wheat was gradually replacing barley. The wheaten cakes kept fairly well after cooking and could be eaten later. This was not possible with barley meal. By this time, the naked wheats, which are more suitable for breadmaking, had largely displaced the husked, or emmer, wheat of earlier times. It is likely that emmer wheats had been used to make unleavened bread, especially for ritual occasions, and the husking was probably effected by burning off the ears. This process is suggested by the sentence in the Bible in the Book of Ruth, which refers to 'parched corn'.

By Graeco-Roman times both a hard and a soft wheat had been developed, the latter making the most palatable bread. But the process was time-consuming and expensive, so that the result, white bread, was a luxury reserved only for the rich. At the same time a coarse wholemeal bread was made, which had known laxative properties. Since it would be inhospitable to offer such bread to guests, wealthy people of high social status served their guests with bread made from fine flour, and white bread became a status symbol. It was probably produced by sieving a well-ground wheaten flour, which separated the flour from the bran and the sand that had been added to the grind mix to help remove the husks.

With the expansion of the Roman Empire wheaten bread

became the staple cereal food in the Mediterranean area, and this Roman preference was to persist throughout Europe for over 2,000 years. In England, for example, in A.D. 1206, the *Assize of Bread* was established to prevent speculation in flour and excessive fluctuations in the price of bread. The legislation laid down how millers' and bakers' charges and the retail price of bread should vary with the cost of the grain. The usual bread was made from wheat, although rye and other cereals were grown, mainly to provide food for animals. Barley was grown principally for brewing beer, although it was eaten by the poor. In other northern European nations rye bread was as important a food as wheaten bread. But even in those countries, the richer families chose white wheaten bread.

For five hundred years the Bread Assizes in England controlled the price of bread, recognizing three grades: white, wheaten, and household. The white flour was reserved for the feudal families, and was baked in small loaves (like dinner rolls) weighing about 200 g each. They were soft in texture and white in colour. The lesser gentry ate a loaf weighing about 500 g, which was made of whole wheat from which the coarse bran had been sieved. The poor and the servants ate a coarse loaf in which wheat wholemeal, rye, and barley flour were mixed. This was known as household bread. The long period during which bread was graded and controlled confirmed in the minds of the English that white bread was a superior food, softer and more palatable, and with the rise of the mercantile classes it became a status symbol to have white bread on the table. There was also a belief that wholemeal bread caused diarrhoea, and diarrhoea could be lethal, especially in children. People probably confused the laxative effects of wholemeal bread with the deadly symptoms of typhoid and other enteric diseases. The third reason was that wholemeal bread resembled oatmeal, which was eaten by the despised Scots. The poor of England also rejected potatoes as a substitute for bread, as they were only used for animal feed, and were eaten by the dirty, decadent, Papist Irish.

The belief that white bread was superior to brown, that it was nutritionally better, tasted better, and was to be preferred, was a long-lasting cultural tradition, but despite popular belief, no objective, scientific investigations had been made to confirm or deny the superiority of white bread over brown. Some people dissented from the popular view. They were mostly intellectuals, usually had good incomes, and were generally regarded as cranks. De Quincey, the self-confessed opium addict, perhaps typifies them and their views. In a letter to a friend, inviting him to stay at Wordsworth's house in Grasmere, De Quincey wrote, 'I would offer you some temptations . . . mountain lamb . . . trout and pike . . . bread, such as you have never presumed to dream of, made of our own wheat, not doctored and separated by the usual miller's process into insipid flour, and coarse—that is merely dirty-looking white, but all ground down together, which is the sole receipt of having rich, lustrous, red-brown ambrosial bread.'

To the average Englishman, De Quincey's views were suspect, his prose too ethereal, and his tastes too exotic. What an Englishman and his family wanted was good, fresh, spongy, white bread.

JH, who is otherwise unnamed, wrote a letter as 'Advocate for Public Welfare' in 1773: 'On the occasion of the public enquiry concerning the most fit and proper bread to be assized for general use.' In the letter he wrote, 'The prejudices of the people are strong; but they relate chiefly to the magic of the two syllables *white* and *brown.*'

The magic of these two syllables has persisted until today, but now there is scientific evidence on which to base the decision whether to eat white bread or brown.

The scientific assessment of the nutritive values of brown and white bread remained a dream until 1945 because of the ethical impossibility of performing a feeding experiment on humans. Then, in the aftermath of the most destructive war in history, undernutrition was the lot of many Europeans, particularly Germans. In these circumstances, the Department of Experimental Medicine at Cambridge University suggested to the Medical Research Council that it would be ethically possible to set up an experimental feeding scheme, under the direction of Professor McCance.

In the town of Wuppertal in the state of Westphalia, Germany, there was a home for abandoned children, aged from 5 to

15 years old. In 1947 food was in short supply, and examination showed that the children were shorter and ligher than American children of corresponding ages. In fact they weighed 9 per cent less and were 5 per cent shorter than their American counterparts. The plan was that in addition to the food rations available, the children would be divided into five groups, each of which would be given a different kind of bread. They would be encouraged to eat as much bread as they liked. The five breads were made of wholemeal flour, 85 per cent flour, 70 per cent flour enriched with vitamins and iron to the concentration found in wholemeal, 70 per cent flour with vitamins and iron in the concentration found in 85 per cent extracted flour, and finally, bread made of 70 per cent unenriched flour. The children were carefully examined at the start of the feeding programme, and received supplements of calcium and vitamins A, C, and D throughout the experiment. They were to be examined again from time to time and tested for levels of protein, vitamins of the B complex, and iron, for these nutrients were known to be removed during milling.

Once the breads were available, the children fell on this extra windfall like ravenous wolves. Quite soon they were all getting about 70 per cent of their calories from bread. In addition they had soups, potatoes, and vegetables, but meat and eggs were very scarce, providing only about 8 g of protein a day.

Professor McCance argued that 'with such a high proportion of bread in their diets, and so little protective foods, everything possible had been done to bring out the differences in the nutritional value of the breads', and the differences would show up quite quickly. In fact no differences appeared. The children in each of the five groups began to improve at an equal rate. At the end of the year there were still no differences, but by now the children had heights and weights comparable to their American counterparts.

After this experience, Professor McCance and his colleagues studied other groups of children and also began animal experiments on feeding young rats.

In 1951 and 1954 the results of their work were published in two special reports by the Medical Research Council of Great Britain. These reports made it clear that following the field experiments in feeding German children, and the laboratory experiments feeding rats, it was 'most improbable that nutritional differences between one bread, or another, would ever be demonstrated in children whether they were well-nourished or undernourished', even when the rest of their diet contained only small quantities of milk, animal protein, or other 'protective' foods, such as vitamins and trace elements. But the reports confirmed the importance of having some of the protective foods in every diet.

It seems then, as far as nutrition is concerned, it matters very little whether 'some gave them white bread and some gave them brown'. But nutrition is not the only factor. A further question has to be asked. Does a diet largely consisting of white refined flour, and large additions of refined sugar, have any other effect on health? Until this is answered the choice between wholemeal bread and bread made from lower extractions of meal must remain open.

As far as your *nutrition* is concerned it doesn't matter whether you eat refined or wholemeal bread. As far as your *health* is concerned, wholemeal bread is superior.

Three groups appear to favour white bread. These are the public, the millers, and the bakers. To the general public, white bread still has a status value: when fresh it is spongier, it looks cleaner, and many think it tastes better, even though the taste is often that of a superior cardboard. The millers prefer white flour because they can produce it more cheaply than brown, and by adding improvers (to make the bread still whiter) believe that the public will buy more bread, which makes for higher profits. They also have the 20 per cent residue left after milling. This is the bran that is sold for animal foods, or as the 'medicinal' bran sold in pharmacies. The bakers prefer white bread because it is easier to mould the dough and bake the bread in today's mechanized bakeries.

In opposition are two groups who advocate brown, high-extraction or wholemeal bread. The first and most vocal group today are those who want a return to a more organic type of food, a food on which no chemicals have been used during growth, and no additives have been used in processing. They reject much of the artificiality of modern life, and seek a simpler, more harmonious, existence.

The second group are those who believe, on scientific evidence, that the consumption, over the years, of low-extraction flours and large quantities of refined sugar may damage health. Although they are currently increasingly vocal, their views are not all that new and have been propagated from time to time over the past centuries. Today, however, their beliefs are supported by much more evidence and are held by people in many countries.

A particularly important investigation has been to study the diseases characteristic of modern Western civilization, but almost unknown in the developing countries of Africa, Asia, and Latin America. Dr Denis Burkitt had a long and distinguished career in Africa before returning to England to take up an appointment with the Medical Research Council. Recently he has been studying the effects of fibre in the diet. Fibre is another term for the outer part of plants (the plant wall and certain other substances), which has little or no nutrient value. It is the bran of wholemeal, the fibre of unrefined sugar, and the fibre in vegetables and fruit. Most nutritionists have ignored the fibre content of the diet until recently, because it is indigestible. Now Denis Burkitt and his colleagues question whether this has not been a dangerous error.

Since the last quarter of the nineteenth century very considerable changes have taken place in the British diet. In about 1870 steel rollers replaced the traditional stones for grinding flour. The steel rollers separated the husk from the flour more efficiently than the traditional grinding stones, so that greater quantities of white flour became available at a reduced cost, enabling more people to choose the whiter breads with lower extraction rates. In 1870 an average person ate about 400 g of bread per day. In addition he ate 300 g of potatoes, together with vegetables and a little fruit. This diet yielded about 40 g of dietary fibre, about 8 g of which was crude fibre, mainly from cereals.

Since 1870 the average consumption of bread has fallen to about 250 g a day, and white bread is chosen in place of wholemeal bread. The consumption of potatoes has fallen to 200 g a day. At the same time, much more sugar and fat are eaten.

In 1875 sugar and fat (to a lesser extent) contributed about 20 per cent of a person's daily energy needs, the rest coming mainly from cereals and potatoes. Today sugar and fat (the consumption of which has increased by only 12 per cent in the past century) provides nearly 60 per cent of daily energy needs. Because of these changes, the average amount of dietary fibre eaten each day is about 11 g, of which about 2 g is crude fibre. This means that the diet eaten by most people contains one-quarter of the fibre eaten by people 100 years ago.

One major effect of the change of diet, according to Denis Burkitt, has been to alter the behaviour of our intestinal tracts and to prolong the time it takes for food to pass from entering the mouth to appearing as faeces in the lavatory pan. With the aid of colleagues in South Africa and London, Dr Burkitt examined the transit times of stools in various groups of people eating different diets. To do this, volunteers swallowed 25 radio-opaque pellets the size of rice grains, and collected the next five or six stools, which they passed into plastic bags. By this simple method, the investigators were able to determine how long it took the pellets to pass through the gut, and also to relate the transit time to the size of the stool. The groups of volunteers who ate a refined, low-fibre diet were British naval ratings and their wives, teenage British boarding-school students, and white university students in Africa. The groups who ate a mixed diet, with a moderate amount of fibre, were hospital patients in England, Indian nurses in South Africa, urban African school children, English vegetarians, and Ugandan African boarding-school students. The groups who ate a high-fibre diet were rural school children in South Africa and rural villagers in Uganda.

When the results were analysed, Dr Burkitt found that the more fibre there was in the diet, the bulkier the stool was and the faster the bulky soft stool was propelled through the bowel. This was true whether the person was a rural Ugandan villager, or a vegetarian English vicar. Those who had a high fibre content in their diet had similar bowel habits; the transit time was about 40 hours, and the stool weighed over 300 g. In contrast those people who ate a traditional English diet, with a low fibre and high sugar content, had daily stools weighing about 110 g, and a transit time of 80 hours. It was interesting that when bran was added to the traditional English diet, the bulk of the stool increased nearly to that of the English vegetarian's, and the transit time diminished.

Following Dr Burkitt's work, Dr Payler in Malvern, Worcestershire gave volunteers, whose stool transit times he had measured using radio-opaque markers, additional fibre in the form of miller's bran and wholemeal bread. Each volunteer took two heaped dessertspoonfuls (about 14 g) of bran each day, which contains about 1.5 g of crude fibre, and an average of two slices of wholemeal bread each day. After 22 days on the new diet the stool transit times had fallen from $64\frac{1}{2}$ to 46 hours, and the weight of the stool had increased by 21 per cent. Later work has shown that most of the increased weight is due to water retained in the stool by the bran, and to an increase in solid material.

Dr Burkitt's work, and that of the other investigators, confirms that diets containing the higher amount of fibre result in large quantities of soft stools which pass through the intestine quickly. But the refined low-fibre diets, favoured in the developed nations, produce small, firm stools which linger in the bowel for a long time. No wonder the British are so obsessed with their bowel function, and resort so readily to laxatives!

If this were merely a scientific observation nothing more need be written. But there is more.

A number of diseases seem to be characteristic of developed Western nations but are rarely encountered in the developing countries. One group of these diseases, commonly found in Western civilizations, are bowel diseases. Appendicitis has become a common disease, and although often misdiagnosed, constitutes a very considerable problem. For example, in 1975 over 300,000 cases of appendicitis were reported in the U.S.A. Diverticular disease, which is an irritation or inflammation of portions of the lower part of the large bowel, is even more common, and affects more than one-third of people over the age of 40. Polyps, and other benign tumours of the bowel, which are now diagnosed more frequently, affect over 20 per cent of Western men aged 20 or more. More sinister, cancer of the bowel is diagnosed in more than 75,000 Americans each year, and over 46,000 die each year from the disease. In Britain, 80 people in every 100,000 of the population, a total of over 45,000 people, have ulcerative colitis and suffer from a painful, chronic disease. Hiatus hernia, which is separation of the tissues of the diaphragm, allowing part of the stomach to enter the chest cavity, is being diagnosed with increasing frequency in Britain, Europe, and the U.S.A. Haemorrhoids affect more than a third of all Western adults over the age of 50, making defaecation painful and requiring painful treatment.

Varicose veins are also being diagnosed with greater frequency. It has been estimated in Europe that 10–20 per cent of adults have varicose veins, and in the U.S.A. 12 per cent of adults have the condition. Black and white Americans have the same incidence of the disorder. In contrast, fewer than 5 per cent of black Africans develop varicose veins.

All the diseases mentioned are uncommon in the developing nations, except among the more affluent citizens who have adopted a Western life-style and a predominantly Western diet. Moreover, it is only in the past century that the diseases have become so common in the developed countries. Appendicitis was unusual in Britain before the end of the nineteenth century, and diverticular disease was rare. These diseases became common after the change in diet which, as I have mentioned, occurred in about 1870 and gathered momentum over the next half century, so that today about 15–20 per cent of the total population of a Western nation will have an appendicectomy at some time during their life. It is interesting too, that both appendicitis and diverticular disease were unusual amongst American blacks until two generations ago, at a time when their dietary habits were changing. Among the Japanese in Japan the diseases are unusual, but they are common amongst the Hawaiian Japanese who have been brought up on a Western cereal diet which is high in refined sugar, and low in fibre.

None of this is intended to suggest that diet is the only factor involved. But the evidence supports the hypothesis that altered dietary habits, and particularly the change from wholemeal bread to low-fibre white bread, and packaged breakfast cereals, the change in the type of vegetables and fruit eaten, and the increasing use of refined sugar, have played an important part.

The low fibre and high refined sugar content of today's

preferred diet has led to a small, firm stool which lingers in the bowel for a long period, and in some way alters the environment, or the 'ecology' of the bowel, by changing the physiological processes in the gut and affecting the uncountable bacteria which inhabit it. This has resulted in an increase in man's tendency to develop bowel diseases.

There is a great deal of evidence to show that appendicitis may be due to a raised pressure inside the appendix, which occurs when a nugget of hard faeces impacts in it. The impactation alters the blood flow to the appendix and stops drainage from it. The changed environment stimulates the bacteria which live there to become active, with the result that the appendix becomes infected and inflamed.

The suggestion that the increased frequency of appendicitis is due to environmental factors, particularly dietary ones, is not new. A few scientists have maintained for at least fifty years that the reduced intake of dietary fibre which altered the habits and bacterial flora of the bowel was the main cause. But they were mostly ignored or, more often, attacked for their opinions. In 1939, for example, an authoritative article stated categorically that the influence of 'geography, diet, and culture', on the incidence of appendicitis was 'mythical'.

Times have changed. Today there is increasing evidence that changes in the dietary habits of Western man to a diet which contains less fibre and more refined sugar has been a major cause of the increased incidence of appendicitis. A careful study investigating the prevalence of appendicectomy in South Africa among various ethnic groups by Dr Walker and his colleagues has shown that appendicectomy is very uncommon among black Africans in rural areas, slightly more common amongst Africans living in the towns and among Eurafricans and Indians, but very much more common among Europeans. Dr Walker also observed that the Africans obtain a far larger fibre intake from their diet, have a shorter stool transit time and a greater frequency of bowel action than the Europeans. What is perhaps even more interesting is the study in which Dr Walker compared the dietary habits and prevalence of appendicectomy in European school and university students with those of adolescents of a similar age in 'Homes' to which they had been admitted because of indigence or adverse family circumstances.

The former group ate a diet containing 4 g of crude fibre, the latter a diet containing 7 g of crude fibre, and both groups ate comparable amounts of refined sugar (90 g daily). Yet among the adolescents in the Homes, the appendicectomy prevalence was only one-fifth that of the other group. Dr Walker comments, 'Our findings . . . indicate that the incidence of appendicitis in a Western community can indeed be markedly reduced.' The diet in the Homes, which contained more oatmeal, wholemeal, bread, and maize (which is rich in fibre) but fewer cakes, pastries, sweets, soft drinks, and ice-cream than the diet of the other Europeans, is 'one that could be readily consumed throughout life. In pattern it is the diet of our ancestors a century or so ago.' The evidence from this study shows that once a person changes to this type of diet he rapidly becomes less prone to appendicitis.

The irritable, or irritated, bowel syndrome has become increasingly common in recent years. It particularly affects women in their mid-thirties and later, and has frequently been dismissed as a psychosomatic condition due to sexual frustration or disappointment in marriage, and to the 'suburban blight'. There is some evidence that the condition may be precipitated by diet, and may be a precursor to diverticular disease. If a high-sugar, low-residue diet is eaten over many years, the faeces tend to be small and firm. The intestines contract segmentally in a strong manner in an attempt to move the faeces on; this raises the pressure inside the gut, causing spasms and pain. In 1973, further evidence of the effect of diet on the irritable (or irritated) bowel syndrome was made by Dr Harvey, working in Bristol. He found that the addition of 30 g of bran each day to the diet of healthy volunteers reduced the stool transit times of those whose previous transit times was fast, so that after 4 weeks the stool transit times of all the volunteers was averaging out at 48 hours. In 1977 Dr Manning, who worked with Dr Harvey, observed that if you don't like bran you can eat wholemeal bread. He found that four slices of wholemeal bread were as effective as bran in reducing the symptoms of the irritable bowel syndrome.

From all their observations, Dr Harvey and his colleagues believe that additional fibre in the diet, in some way 'normalizes' bowel behaviour, and that the adoption by Western man of foods made from white flour induces abnormal behaviour of the colon, leading either to sluggish action or to over-activity.

Alternating diarrhoea and constipation, with or without left-sided abdominal pain, are common in the irritated bowel syndrome, and in the more annoying diverticular disease. Perhaps a low-residue diet, eaten over many years, so alters bowel function that it only needs a psychological insult to make the altered function noticeable, in other words to produce disease. Diverticular disease, which tends to occur somewhat late in life and affects both sexes, is thought on good evidence to be the result of raised pressure in the gut caused by faecal delay in the bowel as a result of a low-residue diet. The disease is rare among people who eat a diet containing much fibre, and occurs with increasing frequency, after a time lag of 15 to 20 years, if they change to a low-fibre diet. Recently an English surgeon, Dr Painter, has shown that many if not most cases of diverticular disease can be treated successfully if the patient takes two heaped dessertspoonfuls (about 14 g) of coarse bran each day with his diet. Coarse bran is preferable to 'processed' bran because it retains more water in the gut, which in turn leads to a bulkier stool and a reduced time before the stool is expelled.

The higher incidence of intestinal polyps, bowel cancer, and ulcerative colitis in Western societies is less easy to explain. Once again there is suggestive evidence. Polyps, bowel cancer, and ulcerative colitis are found in the same populations, and if one disease is rare in a community, so are the others. This suggests some common factor in their causation. One opinion is that the conditions result from bowel irritation due to the release of bile acids and salts from the slowly passing, firm, small stools in the bowel by the bacteria which inhabit it.

There is no real agreement among scientists over whether or not this is a factor in bowel cancer.

In 1974 Dr Wynder and his colleagues suggested that a diet rich in fat, eaten over a period of years, may lead to bowel cancer. The evidence he produced supported his theory but subsequent investigations have led to some doubt. For example Danes develop bowel cancer four times as frequently as Finns living in rural areas, but both eat about the same amount, and type, of fat in their diets.

More recently a study group called the International Agency

for Research into Cancer has suggested that lack of fibre in the diet may be a major factor in the development of bowel cancer. The Agency suggests that dietary fibre may protect people from developing bowel cancer, either because of some unknown factor in the fibre itself or because modern low-fibre diets delay the passage of the faeces through the gut. Food which is rich in fats and which moves relatively slowly through the bowel may cause the body to release excessive amounts of bile salts into the gut to break down the fats into smaller particles. The bacteria which normally live in the gut act on the excessive amounts of slowly moving bile salts and break them down. In the process, substances are formed which remain in contact with the gut lining for longer than would occur if the stool passed more quickly through the gut. Some scientists believe that these substances (which for the chemically-minded are related to deoxycholic acid) may promote ulceration of the bowel, the development of polyps and even bowel cancer in susceptible people.

The evidence that this occurs is still circumstantial, but we know that bowel cancer is less common in people who eat more fibre (and less sugar) in their diet than amongst people who eat fibre-depleted diets.

The increased incidence of haemorrhoids, hiatus hernia, and varicose veins amongst Western peoples can also be explained, at least in part, by the altered dietary habits of the past century. The low-fibre diets lead to constipation, which is increasingly common in Britain. To expel a firm, small, constipated stool demands a considerable effort. This is achieved by fixing the diaphragm, taking in a deep breath, and tightening the abdominal muscles. The result is that the intra-abdominal pressure is raised to an astonishing degree. This increase is repeated until eventually the stool is expelled, or the struggle is abandoned for that day.

Each time the abdominal pressure is raised, the pressure increases in the three 'cushions' of veins and muscle which lie just inside your anus and which assist in keeping the faeces inside your bowel until you want to defaecate. The result of repeated efforts to expel a firm, constipated stool raises the pressure in the veins, which eventually dilate because their walls are unable to cope with the strain. These dilated veins

become varicosities and often prolapse. The result is haemorrhoids, or piles.

One of the factors leading to varicose veins may be the way
in which we empty our bowels. In contrast to the majority of the
people in the world, we sit rather than squat when we defaecate. When you squat to defaecate the direction of the force of
the raised intra-abdominal pressure is down into your pelvis
directly along the line of the lowest portion of your gut. When
you sit to defaecate much of the force is transmitted down your
legs, raising the pressure within your leg veins.

Your leg veins have valves in them to prevent such pressure
causing harm, but if these valves are not very efficient, or are
constantly put under pressure, they may stretch, leading to
increased pressure in the veins and later distension of the veins
themselves. Varicose veins develop.

It is interesting to observe that societies who eat a traditional
diet which contains a good deal of fibre rarely suffer from
varicose veins: fewer than 2 per cent of the adult population are
affected. However, in the affluent nations between 10 and 20
per cent of adults have varicose veins.

A diet rich in sugar and based on low-fibre (refined) cereals,
which leads to a slow transit of the stool and greater difficulty in
defaecation, seems a likely cause of the increased prevalence of
varicose veins in Western societies, although it is probably not
the only cause.

The effect of the raised intra-abdominal pressure, upwards,
not downwards, may account for the increase in hernias of the
diaphragm. These are called hiatus hernias. Hiatus hernia is an
uncomfortable disorder which becomes increasingly common
with advancing age. In affluent, overfed countries routine
barium meal examinations have shown that about 20 per cent of
men and 35 per cent of women have the condition. In the
hungry developing nations, whether the country is Nigeria,
Tanzania, Uganda, India, or Iraq, the number of cases found
has varied from 1 per 1,000 to 1 per cent of the people examined.
This difference is quite astonishing.

The cause of hiatus hernia seems to be the same as that which
leads to haemorrhoids. A low-fibre, high-sugar diet leads to
constipation and to straining when trying to open the constipated bowel. It has been estimated that straining to evacuate a

constipated bowel puts the pressure inside the abdominal cavity up to very high levels. The unnaturally high pressure may be
an important cause of hiatus hernia. And in England, where
women tend to be more constipated than men, the higher
frequency of the disease amongst women could be explained by
this observation.

The prevention and possible treatment of the disease is to
make sure that the diet contains sufficient fibre, and, if it
doesn't, to add bran to the diet, and to make sure that the bowel
is opened regularly.

The relationship between the three common diseases—diverticular disease, appendicitis, and varicose veins—has been
established in a careful investigation by Dr Latto and his colleagues in Reading. Among patients with diverticular disease,
73 per cent also had varicose veins, compared with only 33 per
cent of 'controls'—that is, people of similar age and sex who had
no diverticular disease. And 35 per cent of the patients with
diverticular disease had previously had an appendicectomy.

Dr Latto's findings suggest that the cause of the three conditions is related, and that in susceptible people diet may cause
any one or all of the diseases.

**Many diseases of modern 'civilization', especially hiatus
hernia, appendicitis, diverticular disease, 'irritable bowel',
haemorrhoids, and varicose veins are largely due to our habit
of eating 'refined carbohydrates'—white bread, biscuits, and
sugar, rather than wholemeal flour products.**

The list could go on. But enough has been written to suggest
that the change in our diet, in the past century, to one in which
the high-fibre cereals, such as wholemeal bread, have been
replaced by much smaller quantities of refined flour products
such as white bread, cakes, and breakfast cereals, and much
larger quantities of sugar, have played a part in the diseases of
civilization which affect us. These are constipation, appendicitis, diverticular disease, bowel tumours, haemorrhoids, varicose veins, and hiatus hernia. In all of them, a causative factor is
that the modern diet produces a small, firm, slow-transit stool.
Experiments have shown that constipation can be cured, not

only by laxatives, which stimulate bowel activity artificially, but also adding as little as 2 g of cereal fibre to the diet in the form of unprocessed bran, provided the patient is also willing to regain a normal bowel habit. Since at least £9 million is spent in Britain each year on laxatives, it would seem a great saving in money and a great reduction in suffering if people changed from a diet low in fibre to one high in fibre. In other words, if the British ate wholemeal bread in preference to white bread, cakes, and breakfast cereals, constipation would cease to be the English disease!

'Fibre' in your diet improves your health, and it is cheap—far cheaper than going to your doctor and being prescribed drugs.

However, a diet consisting almost entirely of wholemeal bread is not without certain dangers. In the Punjab in India, for example, the bulk of the diet is made up of unleavened wholemeal bread in the form of chapattis. Susceptible children in the Punjab develop rickets, and in adults a thinning and weakening of the bones occurs. These then become twisted and bent. This condition is termed osteomalacia (or thin bones) and is more often found in women. The two diseases are due to the ingestion of large quantities of wholemeal cereal, and the avoidance of sunshine.

Wholemeal cereal and brown rice contain quantities of a substance called phytate as well as fibre. Phytate and fibre interfere with the absorption of calcium, iron, and zinc from the gut by combining with these minerals. The degree of interference is related to individual sensitivity, but it does constitute a problem when the bulk of the diet is made of wholemeal cereal. In childhood, calcium deficiency may cause rickets, and in adults it may cause osteomalacia. A deficiency of zinc may be a factor in the reduced height and the poor development of the sexual organs, which is fairly common in some West Asian countries.

The average diet of people in the developed nations provides enough extra calcium in dairy foods, such as milk and cheese, and sufficient zinc in protein-rich foods such as meat, to counteract the effects of phytate, should wholemeal cereal be eaten. But when a balanced diet is not eaten, reliance on wholemeal bread, unless calcium, iron, and zinc have been added, may lead to malnutrition, and the appearance of disease.

A balanced view and a balanced diet are needed. The evidence given in this chapter suggests that wholemeal bread should be eaten in preference to white bread (whether this is 'fortified' with calcium and vitamins or not) and, in general, cakes made of white flour should only be eaten occasionally. If you choose to eat white bread because of its softer and spongier texture, its better keeping qualities, and its social status, you should make sure that you eat two heaped dessertspoonfuls of coarse bran (this is about 14 g), or bran crispbread, each day. Fibre is also obtained from fruit (particularly if you eat the skin) and green vegetables, so that you should eat more of these foods. This diet will help you to avoid the bowel and vascular diseases which are becoming increasingly common in Western societies.

Two comments must be added. You won't change the bowel habits of a lifetime overnight. If you are constipated or have bowel symptoms, such as 'gas', belching, nausea, a feeling of abdominal distension, or passing excessive wind, you won't be cured in a week. The beneficial effect of higher fibre in your diet takes weeks or even months to reach its peak. So persist!

As well as this, if you are unused to bran crispbread or to bran itself you have to be careful to begin with. If you eat too much bran in the first two weeks you may find that your stomach gets distended and that you become flatulent. So when you start only take two teaspoonfuls of bran twice daily for three days, then increase this to two teaspoonfuls three times a day—which will give you about 12 g of bran a day. After this, increase the amount each day, if you need to, until you can open your bowels each day without straining. The effect is not immediate, but increases with time over about 12–16 weeks.

Even with this addition to your diet, there is no guarantee that you will avoid bowel diseases. But you will at least stand a better chance of doing so if you choose brown, wholemeal bread, or bran, instead of white bread or plum cake!

4

A sweet but deadly addiction

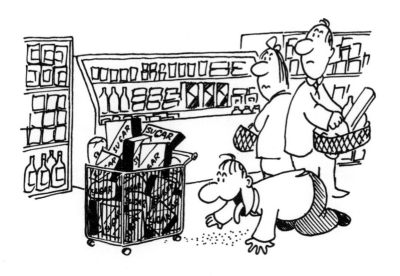

'What are little girls made of?
What are little girls made of?
Sugar and spice and all things nice:
That's what little girls are made of.'
                              Nursery rhyme.

The consumption of refined sugar, usually sucrose, has risen spectacularly in the past 170 years. In Britain in the early 1800s a person ate 25 kg of sugar per year; by 1970 an average person was eating over 50 kg per year. In the U.S.A. the rise in consumption of sucrose has been similar, but slightly lower, so that today in Britain and the U.S.A. between 15 and 20 per cent of the energy value of the diet is provided by sucrose. Sucrose is a carbohydrate, but it is only one source of carbohydrate in food. Unlike cereals, which are made up mainly of the carbohydrate starch, but which also contain protein and other nutrients, sucrose is pure carbohydrate. If it is eaten in addition to the other carbohydrate foods it will almost certainly lead to obesity. Sucrose, or sugar, has been described as being made up of 'empty calories'. The implication is that although sugar provides easily assimilated calories, it contains no other nutrients and if it replaces more complex carbohydrate foods the diet will be less nutritious.

Sugar is the only food eaten by man which supplies absolutely no nutrients whatsoever. There is a myth that because sugar is 'pure energy', the calories are absorbed into the blood (as glucose and fructose) more quickly than other carbohydrate calories. Statistically, it is true that if, for example, you eat sucrose instead of a piece of bread, the sugar enters the bloodstream fractionally more quickly from the sucrose, but in practical terms the difference is so small that it has no noticeable effects. In fact, an athlete 'needing energy' (which is again a doubtful concept, since he uses stored energy in any case) could just as usefully eat a piece of bread as suck a sugar cube.

Sugar contains only 'empty calories'; it contains no protein, fat, vitamins, or minerals.

Nor is there any truth in the belief of health faddists that only white refined sugar lacks nutrients. 'Raw' sugar is just as devoid of nutrients as white sugar. Both consist of 'empty calories'. Refined sugar is 99.9 per cent pure sucrose; raw sugar contains

96 per cent sucrose, 1 per cent water, and 3.3 per cent fibre and molasses. The advantage of eating raw sugar is not that it is nutritionally better, but because of its fibre and its rather different flavour people tend to eat less of it.

As nations, and individuals, become more affluent and economically 'developed', the diet changes. People in affluent countries eat more animal protein, more saturated fat, more total fat and more sucrose than the poor people of the world. They obtain most of the extra fats and sucrose from prepackaged 'convenience' foods and from sugar-rich drinks, and they eat fewer complex carbohydrates (or starches) obtained from cereals, grains, and vegetables, preferring instead to eat refined white flour. In contrast the diet of people in the hungry, economically developing nations consists mainly of complex carbohydrates, fruits, and vegetables, with small amounts of animal protein and fats on feast days.

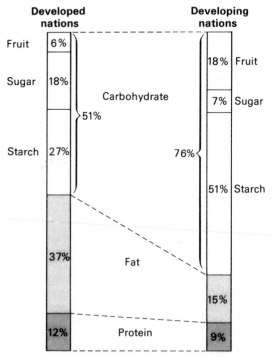

Composition of adult diet in the developed and the developing nations

The changed pattern of diet in affluent nations, particularly the increased consumption of sugar, is especially marked among children and teenagers.

In this vulnerable group up to 50 per cent of the calories eaten each day is supplied by sugar. In the U.S.A., according to the U.S. Agricultural Service, children aged 12–14 are the greatest sugar eaters. In 1969, boys of this age ate 49 g of sugar a day, that is 17.9 kg of sugar a year! Girls ate rather less. They only ate 43 g of sugar a day, or 15.7 kg a year. In Britain Professor John Yudkin found that teenage boys (aged 15–19) ate 156 g of sugar a day or 57 kg a year, while teenage girls ate only half that amount, 96 g a day or 35 kg a year. From the age of 20 the amount of sugar eaten diminished but, at all ages, the amount English people ate was three times greater than that eaten by Americans.

There is a difference between the type of sugared confectionery eaten in Britain and that eaten in the U.S.A. In Britain the largest amount of the sugar is eaten in the form of 'sweets', or as chocolate (which contains fat as well). The second largest amount of sugar is eaten in cakes and biscuits. The degree to which English confectionery preferences are reinforced by advertising is shown by the fact that in 1967 the expenditure on television advertising for sweets and chocolates was the highest for any single product and was 5 per cent greater than the extremely high expenditure for advertising detergents. In Australia a similar situation exists.

In the U.S. the greatest consumption of manufactured sugar is in the form of ice-cream, and Americans only spend about half as much per head on sweets as the British. However, Americans enjoy sweet foods, and sucrose is added to foods as diverse as tinned soups and baked beans.

Why do people in affluent nations eat so much sugar? And is there any harm in it? The answer to the second question will become clear in this chapter. The answer to the first question is, of course, crucial if habits are to be changed but is, alas, speculative.

Sugar, because it is sweet, helps form our concept of what is palatable in food. Palatability is defined as those subjective qualities of food: its texture, its colour, its taste, and its smell or absence of smell. Pure white sugar looks good, it has a good clean texture, and, most important of all, it tastes good! Taste preferences are probably not inborn, but learned. From our earliest childhood days we are given sugar.

Most people living in the rich developed world are addicted to sugar.

Today most babies in the developed nations are bottle-fed, and mothers usually add sucrose to the feed rather than the more appropriate lactose. Young children are rewarded for being good by being given sweets, toffees, chocolate biscuits, or cakes. A woman is brainwashed by advertising to feel that she is a poor mother, a bad wife, and an inadequate homemaker unless she bakes cakes for her children. Children take snacks of sweets to school and school tuck-shops make most of their money by selling sweets, lollies, chocolates, cakes, and soft drinks. All these foods contain sucrose. And it is this pattern of eating that leads the average person in Britain to eat 140 g of sugar (5 oz) a day and the average American to eat 124 g (4¼ oz) a day. Oddly, most people have no idea how much sugar they eat each day because most of it is hidden in manufactured foods. In the U.S.A. only 36 per cent of the total daily intake of sugar, that is, 45 g (1½ oz), is eaten in the form of sugar put on cereals, on fruit, or in tea and coffee. In England the proportion of household sugar is 58 per cent (81 g or 3 oz). The rest consists of the sugar which has been added to manufactured foods.

It is hidden sugar which we don't know we are eating. But we will not stop eating sugar. We have become addicted. Our taste buds have become addicted. We like the taste of sweet things. And because we are addicted, food manufacturers and processors go out of their way to pander to our addiction by adding sugar to many foods. To too many foods!

Professor Yudkin believes with considerable justification that sugar, particularly sucrose, is 'pure, white, and deadly'.

Disturbing information about the effects of feeding very small infants with too much carbohydrate, either in the form of giving them cereals unduly early in life, or especially of adding extra sugar to milk and to 'baby cereals' has been reported from

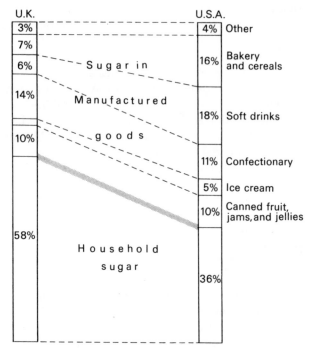

Sugar eaten in the home in the U.K. and the U.S.A.

Scandinavia and Britain and has been discussed in Chapter 1. It appears that the excess of carbohydrate is rapidly converted into fat (which is the normal process), and this fat is stored in fat cells which have to be made to cope with the demand for storage. As I discussed in Chapter 1, the extra fat cells increase the chance of the individual becoming obese, as appetite is determined in part by habit, and in part by the number of fat cells in the body. So fat infants tend to become fat children and to grow into fat adults. And these fat adults find it very difficult to lose weight. They usually remain obese. Obesity is a health hazard, and adult obesity may have been 'programmed' by a mother overfeeding her baby from very soon after birth with additional cereal solids (to which sugar is usually added) and by adding cane or beet sugar—that is, sucrose—rather than milk sugar or lactose to the infant's feeds. From this it follows that coronary heart disease, higher insurance premiums, job problems, and the chance of dying prematurely may all begin when a mother overfeeds her infant by giving it more refined carbohydrate, more cereal, and more sugar than it needs. She is killing it with misplaced kindness.

As the infant grows and becomes a child and later an adolescent, his sugar addiction increases. An investigation by a group of dental surgeons of 2,300 13-year-old children living in Dundee showed that each child, on average, gobbled 500 g (17½ oz) of sweets and chocolates each week. The child eating the least amount managed to eat through 170 g or 6 oz, and the champion sweet eater managed nearly 1,000 g or 35 oz of confectionery in a week!

Sugar addiction is well established by adolescence and has two unpleasant effects. One of them is aggravation of dental caries, and the other is aggravation of diabetes in susceptible people.

Dental caries is one of the penalties of affluence and of an unsuitable diet. A careful investigation in 1952 by the U.S. National Research Council could find no evidence that ancient man suffered greatly from dental caries, and today it is rare among primitive tribes who have avoided the persuasiveness of traders or missionaries. In England in 1960 a dental surgeon, Professor Hardwick, examined over 1,000 teeth in skulls which carbon-dating had established belonged to people who were living in about the sixth century of the Christian era. He compared them with a similar number of modern teeth. Dental caries had occurred in only 9.5 per cent of the Anglo-Saxon teeth, but was present in 48.6 per cent of modern teeth. In fact, dental caries is now so common that it might be considered normal. Surveys in Britain show that by the age of 18, an average of 5 teeth have decay. Similar surveys in the U.S.A. and Australia indicate that by the age of 20 an average of 15 teeth are carious, and 5 teeth have been extracted. As adult humans have 32 permanent teeth, this means that by the age of 20, 47 per cent of the teeth are decaying, and 16 per cent have been extracted. A survey in Australia has also revealed that by the age of 20, one person in five wears false teeth.

In these surveys, and in the more intensive investigations

made of small groups of teenagers, it has been found that the more sugar that is eaten *between* meals, especially if it is eaten in the form of sweets, caramels, or toffees, the greater the incidence of subsequent caries. But if the sugar is only eaten *with* meals the high incidence of caries does not arise.

It has also been found that fluoride, added to drinking water, to some extent protects against tooth decay induced by addiction to sugar. Fluoride hardens the tooth enamel, preventing its erosion by the acids produced by the interaction of sucrose and the millions of bacteria that live in the mouth.

There is no doubt that dental disease has become more common in the past 150 years as man has eaten more and more sugar. But the connection between sugar and dental caries was noted by an observant German traveller to England as long ago as 1598. He remarked on the black teeth of Queen Elizabeth and on his return to Germany suggested that this was 'a defect the English seem subject to from their too great use of sugar'.

The relationship between sugar intake and dental caries is also supported by observations made in several countries during and after the Second World War, when sugar was rationed. Although people were able to obtain less sugar, their total consumption of carbohydrates increased. What they did was to substitute bread, flour, potatoes, and vegetables for sucrose. Sweets, manufactured biscuits, and cakes were rationed, so children were given 'treats' of fruit instead, and snacks between meals were eaten much less often.

Observations in Britain, Scandinavia, and Japan, showed that in each of these countries there was a steady, progressive decline during those years in the number of young children who had decaying teeth. But after 1948, when sugar became freely available once again, the prevalence of dental caries began to increase.

Two investigations made in Scandinavia are even more conclusive. In the first, a sucrose-free diet was devised and eaten by a group of children. After a year their dental hygiene was compared with that of a group of children who ate sucrose sweets between meals. The children whose diet contained sucrose had an annual rate of dental caries 8–10 times higher than those who did not eat any sucrose. In the second experiment, two groups of children ate a diet that was normal in every way except that one group ate no sucrose, using instead a sweetener called xylitol. At the end of one year the children's teeth were examined. Those eating the diet with sucrose had developed 5 carious teeth, while those eating the diet without sucrose had one or no carious teeth.

It seems that sucrose is the culprit. Because of the difficulties of carrying out experiments on humans, scientists have turned to animals to investigate whether it is really sucrose and not some other element in the human diet that causes tooth decay.

Luckily, from the point of view of science (if not from that of the animals), certain strains of rats and hamsters are particularly susceptible to dental caries. In an experiment devised by Drs Green and Hartles in Liverpool, various carbohydrate diets were fed to the animals. They found that if the diet contained 70 per cent of raw, uncooked starches derived from wheat, maize, and potato, none of the animals developed dental caries. If the animals were fed partly cooked starchy foods, a few animals developed tooth decay, but if the diet contained 70 per cent sucrose, a high proportion of animals developed dental caries. If the sucrose in the diet was replaced by the simpler sugars, such as glucose, fructose, or maltose, caries still occurred but not to the degree it occurred if the diet contained a high proportion of sucrose.

The experiments confirm that sucrose in the diet does cause dental caries. Why should sugar, whether eaten as sweets or in cakes and biscuits, cause tooth decay? Dental surgeons have worked on this problem and have an answer.

A tooth is mainly made up of a tough bone called dentine, over which is a thin coat of enamel, which is the hardest tissue in the body. Inside the dentine is the tooth pulp which contains nerves and blood vessels. Dental decay begins when particles of food containing sugar stick on to the surface of the teeth, or become impacted into the normal crevices of the tooth's structure. The food particles, together with saliva and the myriads of bacteria that are always in your mouth, form a small plaque, rather like a miniature cow-pat, which sticks tightly on to the tooth's surface. There are two main kinds of bacteria in the plaque. They are called streptococci and lactobacilli. The streptococci convert any sugars in the food (but preferentially convert sucrose) into a complex carbohydrate substance called dextran. The dextran is relished by the lactobacilli, which release an acid as they grow and multiply. The acid is produced in the plaque of food as it adheres to the tooth, and since it is not neutralized by the alkaline saliva, gradually eats into the dentine through cracks in the enamel.

If the diet or the drinking water contains a reasonable amount of fluoride, the dental enamel is less likely to be damaged if a plaque forms on it. Similarly, if the teeth are cleaned after eating snacks, or if snacks are avoided, plaques cannot form so easily and acid build-up is prevented.

But the problem is how to change people's habits, particularly when infants are given sucrose in milk feeds (rather than lactose, which is less sweet but just as much an energy supplier); when small children are rewarded for being good by being given a sweet, a toffee, a biscuit, or a piece of cake; and when school tuck-shops persist in selling sweets and lollies to older children and to adolescents. The problem has not yet been solved, and to understand it needs some thought about what happens when you eat a meal.

When you eat a meal consisting mostly of carbohydrate, and particularly when you eat a meal which is rich in sugar, a sequence of events occurs. The purpose of this sequence is to enable you to absorb the carbohydrate quickly and efficiently, and to transfer it to your liver and muscles where it is converted into the stored form of carbohydrate, glycogen. It is then available to meet the varying energy needs of your body when the demand arises.

The sequence of events is not completely understood, but recent research has given scientists a good deal more knowledge about what goes on, and especially what happens to the body if diabetes develops.

The starches in your food begin to be broken down into sugars (resembling sucrose) in your mouth by the action of your saliva. This process continues in your small intestine where the simpler sugars formed from the starch and the sucrose you have eaten are absorbed into the soft, fine, brush-like surface of the cells covering the inner lining of the intestine. There the sugars are converted into even simpler sugars, of which glucose and fructose are the most common and the most important. Glucose and fructose are absorbed into your blood-stream, and the level of glucose in your blood rises. This in turn provokes a response. Special beta cells in the pancreas (a gland lying close to the intestine) secrete a hormone called insulin. In response to the challenge of rising levels of glucose in the blood, the level of insulin in the blood rises as the beta cells secrete more and more. The greater the glucose challenge, the greater the insulin response. Insulin has the effect of rapidly lowering the high level of glucose in the blood, which occurs just after a meal, to a more normal level. It does this by stimulating complex enzyme systems to convert the glucose into the storage substance glycogen. This action takes place in your liver, and to a lesser extent in your muscles. But insulin has many other equally important functions. It enables body cells to utilize the available glucose more easily, and it prevents the liver from converting glycogen into glucose, so that the body stores of energy remain filled. It also helps in the conversion of glucose into fat, which is a very convenient method of storing energy. This is not all. Insulin also stimulates muscles to produce protein.

The importance of insulin in all these functions is shown in diabetic people. Diabetes is a disease in which the beta cells of the pancreas are unable to produce any insulin or, more usually, produce insufficient insulin to cope with the carbohydrate challenge that occurs when glucose is absorbed into the blood-stream from the gut. In many cases of diabetes the person has inherited a susceptibility to the disease.

Because of the poor response by the cells of the pancreas in producing insulin, the level of glucose in the blood remains high for a long period of time and some of the glucose leaks through the kidney into the urine. This is a classic symptom of diabetes.

It is thought that the insulin-producing beta cells of the pancreas are of two types. The first type of cells have insulin ready for release when the carbohydrate challenge occurs and when the level of glucose in the blood rises. The second kind of insulin-producing cells manufacture and store insulin. As soon as the first type of cells have discharged their content of insulin into the blood, the storage cells transfer insulin into the front-line cells. However, the transfer takes some time.

In very severe diabetes—the kind that usually starts in childhood—both kinds of insulin-producing cells are affected and almost no insulin is produced. Unless children with this defect are given injections of insulin they will become thin (because the fat-depositing effect of insulin is absent) and their muscles will waste away (because the protein formation effect of insulin is absent). As well as this tiny blood vessels in their muscles, in their eyes, and in their kidneys become damaged, so that the children soon die. With injections of insulin and a careful diet the devastating damage of juvenile diabetes can be avoided and the children can live a reasonably normal life.

In the milder form of diabetes, which doesn't usually appear until middle age, only the front-line cells are affected, so that some insulin is released in response to the glucose challenge. But with advancing years the amount released becomes less and less and eventually diabetes develops.

It has been estimated that about one adult in every seven, or 15 per cent of the adult population of Britain, Switzerland, and West Germany have some degree of inadequate response to a glucose challenge and 1–3 per cent will become diabetic by the age of 26. It is likely that similar proportions would be found in other rich overfed parts of the world if surveys were carried out. Evidence from the U.S.A. is even more disturbing. Surveys there have shown that diabetes is being diagnosed more frequently each year. In fact, the incidence is increasing at about 6 per cent each year. If this goes on, twice as many people in the U.S.A. will have diabetes 15 years from now as have the disease today.

Those people who do become diabetic in adult life are usually fat. This suggests that in some way obesity and diabetes are connected. Obesity usually occurs because people over-eat the wrong kinds of food. Over the years people who become fat have eaten too much refined carbohydrate, sugar, and fat.

What then is the connection between diet and diabetes? Is there a connection? It seems there is, although it is less strong in the case of the type of diabetes which starts in childhood, than in the type of diabetes which begins in adult life. Even in the childhood diabetes, diet seems to play a part, and a diet which is low in fibre and high in sugar and refined carbohydrates may be the 'trigger'.

In Britain, over 5,000 children born in 1946 have been examined at intervals ever since that date. Up to the time they were 8 years old, the only flour available in Britain was National flour, which had a relatively high fibre content; but after that date white flour with a low fibre content was re-introduced. In 1957, when the children were aged 11, only one child was found to be a diabetic, an incidence of 0.2 per 1,000. (In 1972, by which time the men and women were aged 26, the prevalence had risen to 3.0 per 1,000.)

Another group of 15,500 children, all born in 1958, have also been studied in a similar manner. These children appear to have eaten rather more sugar than the group born in 1947, and throughout their lives have only eaten low-fibre white flour. In 1969 these children were aged 11. An investigation showed that eight of them (0.5 per 1,000) had diabetes.

Despite these observations, it appears that severe diabetes starting in childhood is almost as common in the hungry developing nations as it is in the rich developed nations. This suggests that the prevalence (that is, the frequency in the community) of the genetic defect is similar in all parts of the world and that diet plays a smaller part in 'triggering' the disease when it starts in childhood (juvenile diabetes).

The relationship between diet and diabetes starting in adult life is much stronger.

Investigations into the diets of many middle-aged diabetics have shown that for several years before the onset of the disease their food intake has been excessive. Their diets have contained an excess of all foodstuffs, but the excess of refined carbohydrate, and especially of sugar, seems to have been of the greatest importance.

Dr Campbell, a diabetic expert, has written, 'Anyone who puts sugar in his tea and drinks five cups a day stimulates his islet (insulin-producing) cells unnecessarily and in a brutal fashion over 91,000 times in 50 years.' And it is certainly true, as I have shown earlier in this chapter, that many people living in the rich developed nations are addicted to sugar. Dr Campbell also believes that the refined carbohydrate used to make bread, cakes, and biscuits which are habitually eaten by most people in the affluent nations, and which I discussed in the last chapter, adds to the insult given to a person's pancreas. He has evidence that refined carbohydrate (from which the dietary fibre has been stripped) is absorbed more rapidly and creates a larger, quicker surge of glucose in the blood. Although the surge is less than that following a sugar meal it is sufficient to provoke the insulin-secreting cells in a 'brutal' manner.

However, it also seems clear that unless you are one of the 15 per cent of the population whose insulin release becomes inadequate with age, obesity is unlikely to provoke diabetes. Unfortunately, there is no test at present that will identify whether you are one of these people early enough for you to avoid the disease should you habitually over-eat.

Investigations have also shown that the type of diabetes which first appears in middle age is much more common in rich countries than in the developing nations. The relative rarity of this type of disease in the latter may be due to the fact that the disease does occur in the community but is under-reported because of the shortage of doctors and the disinclination of people to go to a doctor unless they are really ill.

There is some good evidence that this is not the only reason, and that diabetes is, in fact, uncommon in peasant communities who eat a diet which is low in sugar and in refined carbohydrates. The best documented evidence for this comes from Dr Campbell's careful investigations into diabetes in Natal, South Africa, among rural Zulus, urban Zulus, and Indians.

Among the rural Zulus, who worked for a sugar-cane company in northern Natal, but who ate little refined sugar (although they did chew sugar cane) diabetes was rare. But among urban Zulus, who had adopted a Western type of diet as far as sugar and sugar-rich drinks were concerned, diabetes occurred in 1 per cent of those surveyed. Among Indian communities in Natal, diabetes was even more common. Dr Campbell found that of 975 Indians aged 30 or more living in 'barrack' accommodation provided by a sugar-cane growing company, 10 per cent had sugar in their urine.

Of course, sugar in the urine does not mean that a person necessarily has diabetes. To make the diagnosis, blood sugar estimations (after a glucose feed) or blood insulin estimations have to be made. But surveys in Britain, Canada, Germany, Sweden, and the U.S.A. have shown that between one-third and two-thirds of those with sugar in their urine proved on further testing to have diabetes. If these proportions are applicable to the Natal Indians, between 3 and 7 per cent of them will have diabetes, which is a higher prevalence than found in surveys in Europe and the U.S.A.

These observations suggest that diabetes is more likely to appear in susceptible people in middle or in old age if, over the years, they have eaten a diet which has contained a good deal of sugar, especially if the diet also contained a good deal of refined carbohydrate. In contrast, if they eat a diet containing only a small amount of sugar (and unrefined carbohydrate) they may avoid becoming diabetic. In support of this suggestion is Dr Campbell's observation of the relative infrequency of diabetes among Zulus living in the rural areas. Zulu peasants, who rarely develop diabetes, only eat about 8 g of sugar a day, but urban Zulus eat nearly 100 g a day, and develop diabetes almost as frequently as British people. Indians living in India rarely become diabetic. They eat only about 17 g of sugar a day and diabetes occurs in less than 1 per cent of them. In contrast, Indians living in Natal and working in cane-fields eat 140 g of sugar a day and develop diabetes much more frequently.

Dr Campbell has made a further observation. He believes that diabetes will only appear in the susceptible 15 per cent of the population if the excessive sugar intake has been eaten for a number of years. In the first few years when a sugar-rich diet is eaten, diabetes is rare, but as time passes it becomes more common. In fact 20 years of a diet containing a fair amount of sugar seems to be necessary before diabetes will appear in susceptible people.

Why should a sugar-rich diet provoke the appearance of diabetes? Recently Drs Wicks and Jones, who work in Africa, have come up with an explanation. They have found that Africans who eat a rural type of diet, in which maize is the staple, have a poor, rather slow, insulin response to a carbohydrate challenge. Europeans and urban Africans living in Rhodesia who eat a diet containing a fair amount of sugar and a good deal of white bread have a rapid insulin response. Wicks and Jones suggest that perhaps the beta cells in the pancreas become exhausted over the years of having to respond to a diet which has a high amount of sugar and which is eaten for reasons other than hunger. If a quick insulin response is frequently demanded over the years, because sugar is taken in foods and, perhaps worse, is eaten between meals in snacks and 'soft' sugar-rich drinks, the beta cells may become increasingly less efficient. The glucose challenge has been too great and has occurred too often.

It is interesting to note that if the diet is changed so that sugar is cut out, and other carbohydrates are cut down, the diabetes disappears. Dr Wall and his colleagues found this when they put two hundred fat mature-onset diabetics on a diet which limited carbohydrates to 100–150 g a day and stopped all added sugar. After three weeks on this diet the diabetes had disappeared in 80 per cent of the patients, and in two-thirds of them this had been achieved without much loss of weight.

The evidence is pretty strong that mature-onset diabetes, in susceptible people, is provoked by sugar and perhaps refined carbohydrate eaten over many years.

Although it is obvious that many people in affluent societies are addicted to sugar, and by their addiction are spoiling their teeth and increasing the risk of developing diabetes, it would be ridiculous to ban sugar altogether. In the first place, people would rebel: we need to pander to our addiction. Secondly, the substitutes for sugar—the non-nutrient sweeteners such as saccharin and cyclamates are less palatable than sucrose and have potential health hazards.

Thirdly, sugars have valuable preservative properties. Sucrose added to condensed milk, to jams, jellies, and preserves reduces the likelihood of bacterial growth by its moisture-removing effect. Sucrose is not the most efficient sugar preservative: fructose and dextrose, which are both simple sugars, are nearly twice as efficient. However, they are less sweet and not so easily soluble, so manufacturers usually choose the less efficient but cheaper sugar, sucrose. Sucrose is also used in the manufacture of ice-cream, because it enables it to freeze more easily. In the manufacture of beer, sucrose is needed to supply energy for the yeasts which produce the alcohol. In bread- and cake-making, sugar is needed so that the yeast can rapidly produce the carbon dioxide gas necessary for the raising effect that produces the doughy bread which people demand. It also forms a complex with the gluten of the flour. This helps the gluten to expand, so that a light-textured cake or bread is obtained.

Having said this, it is still true that affluent Western man eats too much sugar in the form of sweets, confectionery, and chocolates. He drinks too much sugar by adding sucrose to his tea, coffee, and soft drinks. He compounds all this by an indulgence in biscuits, cakes, and ice-cream. By eating these empty calories he ruins his teeth, he may be adding to the risk of becoming fat, he may bring to light hidden diabetes, and he may be adding to the risk that he will have a heart attack.

'Anyone who puts sugar in his tea or coffee stimulates his insulin-producing cells in an unnecessary and brutal way.'

How can the sweet but deadly addiction to sugar be avoided? Obviously you have to start as early in life as possible, and certainly before the age of four. Mothers, fathers, uncles, aunts, grandparents, and friends should learn that to give sweets, chocolates, crisps, peanuts, and bottled or canned soft drinks to children is not an act of kindness, but is perhaps just the opposite. A sweet tooth is not inborn but acquired. If a child needs a reward for being good, or is given a present to make the giver feel good, let it be fresh fruit or a fruit drink without added sugars. And when you do this remember that among the rural people of the hungry world, who do not habitually eat much sugar, coronary heart disease, dental caries, and sugar diabetes are uncommon!

To some extent you have a free choice—to become or not to become addicted to sugar. But it is not really as free a choice as that. People imitate, and the child who is not allowed sweets and chocolates when his friends have them may feel deprived. People are influenced by emotion rather than reason. Advertising uses this fact to sell products. Last year in many rich, developed, overfed nations, the cost of advertising sweets, toffees, chocolates, cakes, ice-cream, and soft drinks amounted to over 10 per cent of the total retail sales of the products. Already in the most remote villages in Africa, Asia, and Latin America, the local stores advertise and sell that supreme example of Western dietary influence—Coca Cola. Villagers are beginning to be persuaded that this drink, or one of its orange-flavoured imitators, is preferable to their traditional beverages.

Despite the insidious psychological effects of imitation and advertising persuasion, you can limit your addiction to sucrose—if you want to.

This is how you can do it:

● Start by cutting down the number of spoons of sugar you add to your cup of tea or coffee, and over a few weeks cut out all sugar you use in hot drinks. What you are doing is 'desensitizing' your taste buds' demand for a sweet taste.

● If you eat breakfast cereals don't put sugar on them; if you eat porridge, be like the Scots—add salt, not sugar!

● Avoid eating cakes and sweet biscuits, except on special occasions.

● Cut out ordinary soft drinks, drink low-calorie ones instead. They do contain sweeteners, but the amount of cyclamate or saccharin in them is not going to do you any harm.

● Or better, buy citrus fruit and make your own fruit drink instead. The fructose in the fruit will make it sweet enough and you will not need to add additional sucrose.

● If you drink alcohol, choose the lighter (less sugary) varieties of beer and avoid ginger-ale, bitter-lemon, and tonic in your brandy or gin. The first is very sweet; the others seem to be bitter, but in reality are loaded with hidden sugar.

● Stop eating sweets, chocolates, and toffees between meals. If you need to chew something, chew an apple!

● But don't be obsessive. If you want to eat a cake or a piece of chocolate or some ice-cream, or drink a soft drink from time to time, you can!

5

Two valuable minerals

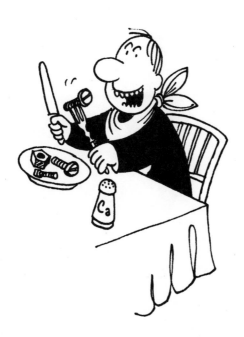

'And your bones are very brittle.'

R. L. Stevenson

Calcium

By the time a person becomes adult he has about 1.2 kg (2½ lb) of calcium in his body. Most of this is in his bones. Calcium is what makes bones hard, and if for any reason the bones lose calcium they become more brittle, fracture more easily, and may even collapse. Those changes occur normally in old age, particularly in women. They occur abnormally in certain younger women who have had their ovaries removed, and in the course of several diseases.

When we are growing up, calcium is steadily absorbed from the diet to supply the needs of the growing bones. Once a person apparently 'stops growing' the amount of calcium in the bones levels off, and remains at 1.2 kg. When the menopause is reached in women, calcium may begin to be lost from bone. Men are not affected in this way until about the age of 65, when they too begin to lose calcium from their bones.

From this you may think that the calcium in the bones, once deposited, is there permanently, rather like the calcium in limestone or chalk. This quite erroneous. Bone is a dynamic structure, constantly being formed and broken down or resorbed. Every day about 700 g of calcium is exchanged between the blood plasma and the bone. Some of this calcium is then excreted in the urine and is lost to the body, but at the same time we obtain calcium from our diet.

An average European diet provides about 1,100 mg of calcium each day, principally in milk and milk products such as cheese, and to a lesser extent in bread (which in England has calcium added to the flour to counteract the calcium-hoarding properties of a substance called phytate). The diet of most people in the hungry developing world does not contain much milk, so that the amount of calcium provided is lower. In India, for example, an average of 350 mg per head per day is obtained, which is only about one-third of that provided by a European diet.

This is not such a serious situation as it might appear. Between 60 and 70 per cent of the 1,100 mg of calcium in the

European diet is not available for absorption, and is lost in the faeces, while a much lower proportion of the calcium in the Indian diet is lost, and more is available to be absorbed.

The calcium is absorbed through the cells lining the intestine by becoming bound to protein-carriers, which transport it from the gut into the blood. Before this can happen there must be a certain amount of vitamin D in the body, as the protein is unable to link to calcium in the absence of this vitamin. When vitamin D is deficient rickets occurs in children and the bones of adults become soft and distorted. This is discussed in Chapter 6.

The calcium is transported in the blood and transferred to the bones or, if the blood level becomes too high, is excreted by the kidneys. Like most other chemical substances, the level of calcium in the blood tends to be maintained within very narrow limits.

Although the limits of the amount of calcium in the blood are strictly regulated, a constant exchange occurs from the calcium in the diet into the blood, from the blood to the bones, from the bones to the blood, from the blood to the kidneys, from the kidneys to the urine, and from the urine back into the blood or out into the lavatory pan.

The regulation of this sequence is complex, and scientists are still discovering more about how it operates. As I mentioned, vitamin D is essential for calcium to be absorbed from the gut.

Once the calcium has been absorbed into the blood-stream the action of vitamin D does not cease. In the blood, the regulation of the level of calcium is controlled largely by a hormone produced by tiny glands which are found in the neck near the thyroid gland. They are called parathyroid glands, and the hormone which they produce is called parathyroid hormone. If the blood level of calcium falls, more parathyroid hormone is secreted. This mobilizes calcium from the bones, and by stimulating vitamin D production in the kidneys reduces the amount lost in the urine.

Provided calcium is being obtained from food, little regulation is required; but at night, particularly, when food is not normally eaten, and when calcium continues to be lost in the urine, parathyroid hormone secretion is increased to maintain the blood level by removing some of the calcium from the bones.

From the description, it might be imagined that a very large amount of calcium would need to be eaten each day, or the bones would lose calcium and become brittle. However, evolution has solved this problem, at least so long as women produce female sex hormones called oestrogens in their ovaries, and men's testicles continue to secrete sex hormones, which are called androgens.

The sex hormones, in some way not yet fully understood, protect the bones from the calcium-extracting action of parathyroid hormone, so that the only way in which the level of calcium in the blood can be maintained is by increasing the amount of calcium the kidneys reabsorb from the urine, and by encouraging the absorption of more of the calcium in the diet.

In most people the system works admirably. The bones, which are constantly being renewed, remain strong and rigid. The diet provides all the calcium needed to keep them strong; there is enough vitamin D to ensure that calcium in the diet is absorbed; and parathyroid hormone regulates the level in the body. But certain things can upset this admirable state of affairs. One is reduced mobility; another is the loss or reduction of the sex hormones.

As people grow older, they become less mobile. They sit about more, or potter about gently, rather than being as active as they were when younger. The most dramatic example of enforced immobility (and weightlessness) was found among astronauts. When the U.S. astronauts returned to earth after a prolonged period in space, it was found that their bones had become demineralized to some degree. They had lost calcium. Once they returned to Earth's gravity and resumed normal activity, the lost calcium was replaced quite quickly.

The loss of sex hormones is unusual in young people except when a woman has to have her ovaries removed or a man has to be castrated. However, after the menopause in women, and rather later in men, the level of sex hormones in the blood falls.

The increased loss of calcium from bones that occurs with age, particularly in the case of women, is related to the reduction in the amount of sex hormones that occurs as people get older. Indeed, several eminent scientists believe that the decalcification of bone which occurs in women after about the age of 50, and in men about 15 years later, is largely due to a deficiency of sex hormones; and the greater immobility of old age is an unimportant factor.

If their views are correct, the loss of bone substance might be expected to affect women earlier, and more severely, than men. Women reach the menopause at about the age of 50. Following the menopause, the level of female sex hormones in their blood falls, as their ovaries no longer produce oestrogens, and the only source of oestrogen is from the adrenal glands and from some areas in the skin. There are, of course, wide variations in the amount of oestrogen produced, but women after the menopause generally have far less than when they were younger. In men, there is no equivalent of the menopause. A man's testicles continue to produce androgens until about the age of 69, after which a slow decline does occur.

When scientists began to study bone density by X-rays, which give a measure of the amount of calcium in the bones, they found that women over the age of 50 had much less dense bones than men of the same age. It was also known from studies in Sweden and in Scotland that women aged 60–70 were five time as likely to break their wrists as women aged 30–40, but in men no such increase occurred. Other physicians had observed that many older women developed severe backache. When X-rayed their vertebrae were seen to be less dense, and occasionally collapsed. This condition is known as osteoporosis, or 'less-dense bones'.

Professor Nordin and his team in Leeds have been investigating osteoporosis for the last 20 years with the help and co-operation of a large number of middle-aged and older women. These volunteers are prepared to go into the laboratory and have various tests made on their blood and urine so that the cause of the disease may be discovered.

Dr Nordin has found that when the level of the female sex hormone oestrogen falls after the menopause, bone formation continues as before, but bone resorption increases. This is because the amount of oestrogen is insufficient to protect the bone against the calcium-removing effect of parathyroid hormone. As you will remember, parathyroid hormone is more active at night, at a time when calcium is not being absorbed from the gut, because none is being eaten.

The loss of calcium from the bones continues slowly and

imperceptibly, only a minute amount being lost each day. But over the years the bones become less dense as their calcium content gets less. Dr Nordin has been able to measure the amount lost by taking X-rays of finger-bones at intervals.

Different bones in the body lose calcium at different rates, and so far scientists have been unable to explain why this happens. The thigh bones are the least affected. In the 10- to 20- year period after the menopause they lose about 5 per cent of the calcium they originally contained. The finger-bones are more affected, and lose about 20–25 per cent of their calcium over the same period. The vertebrae are the most affected and may lose as much as half the calcium they contained in the 10 to 20 years after the menopause. From these statistics it is easy to see why Dr Nordin measured the bone loss in the fingers. They are easy to X ray and to measure, and give the average bone loss when all bones are considered.

The apparent relationship between bone loss and a reduction in sex hormones has led doctors to ask if they could prevent women developing osteoporosis, or at least delay the fractures and the backache, and in the most severe cases, the collapse of a vertebra, by giving female sex hormones to women from the menopause onwards.

The problem is that although some decrease in the calcium content of bones occurs in the years after the menopause, only a few women develop osteoporosis. When they do the usual warning is an acute back pain, which occurs from the partial collapse of a vertebra.

As well as this, the *routine* use of female sex hormones, particularly oestrogens, to protect a postmenopausal woman from osteoporosis (and other diseases) is controversial. Despite a good deal of research, the question has not yet been answered conclusively, but investigations in the U.S.A. and in Scotland on small numbers of women suggest that oestrogens may help to diminish bone loss. There are two snags. The first is that the American doctors found that if a woman took oestrogens for a short period of time—no longer than six months—bone loss was prevented; but if she took the hormone for a longer period of time the bone loss-preventing effect ceased. The Scottish doctors did not find this.

The second problem is that there is grave concern amongst

doctors that oestrogens taken for long periods may predispose the woman to cancer of the womb, to high blood pressure, and possibly to clots in veins.

Because of the possible dangers of oestrogen treatment, I believe it should only be given under strict medical supervision with frequent examinations. But every woman can take measures which will reduce her chances of developing brittle bones if she alters her diet and increases the amount of exercise she takes.

Older women tend to eat a diet containing less milk and cheese than when they were younger, replacing these valuable foods with an increased intake of sweets, cakes, and chocolates. Middle-aged women—that is anyone aged 45 or more—should change to a diet containing at least 0.5 litre (just over 1 pint) of whole or skim milk, and should eat 50 g (1¾ oz) of cheese each day. Half a litre of milk provides 600 mg of calcium; and 50 g of cheese an additional 400 mg. One gram of calcium is usually more than enough to compensate for the loss of calcium in your urine, your faeces, and your sweat. This averages only 400 mg of calcium a day. If people do not like milk but like cheese, they can eat twice the amount of cheese, and the reverse applies if they don't like cheese. And, of course, the milk need not be drunk as milk. It can be taken in drinks, in junkets, and in sauces. The calcium content of milk remains the same irrespective of its food form. Since extra calcium seems to be lost from the bones at night by most menopausal women, it would be wise to drink a glass of milk on going to bed at night. In fact, a group of London scientists have advised postmenopausal women to take in addition a couple of calcium tablets in the late evening, so that between 800 and 1,000 mg of elemental calcium is eaten. They believe that this will prevent the parathyroid hormone removing calcium from bone during the night.

As well as this, postmenopausal women should take exercise. It need not be too strenuous, but should be regular. Walking or gardening are as useful as cycling or playing golf. These measures are simple and safe and not particularly controversial.

Soon we may have more knowledge to provide the answers to the puzzles of calcium metabolism in the body.

Iron

If women are disadvantaged compared with men in their need for calcium, they are even more disadvantaged in their need for iron.

Iron is essential for life. It plays a central role in enabling living cells to obtain the energy they need. In humans iron forms a complex with a substance called haem and a protein. The product, haemoglobin, is formed in the red blood cells of the body, and acts as the vital carrier of oxygen from the lungs to the tissues and cells. The lungs absorb oxygen from the breathed air into the blood. The oxygen is rapidly taken into the red blood cells, where it combines with the haem to form a stable compound. In this way it is safely transported to the cells of the body to supply their energy needs. Once the oxygen is released from the red blood cells and enters the cells of the tissues, another iron-containing substance—an enzyme—is needed so that the oxygen can release its contained energy. Without iron none of this could happen. Yet the human body contains only about 4 g or ¼ oz of iron—the amount contained in a large nail. Three-quarters of the body's iron is in haemoglobin; a small amount (about 5 per cent of the total iron) is held in body cells, and the balance is stored in special cells found mainly in the liver, the spleen, and in bone marrow. This stored iron is available if new supplies are not available from the food, so that the body has a reserve of the vitally needed iron. The reserve is needed because the human body cannot manufacture iron. Man has to obtain the iron he needs from the food he eats or from his mother. The newborn baby starts life with about 300 mg of iron which it has accumulated from its mother during pregnancy. From then on, all the iron it needs must come from its food. In the first few months of life, it gets little iron from the milk it drinks, but when the infant starts eating cereals and other foods it begins to absorb more each day than it loses, so that by the time the child has grown to become an adult its body contains about 4 g of iron.

Each day about 1 mg of iron—the amount in a pinch of salt—is lost in the cells which are shed from your skin, or your gut, or your hair. But each day iron is absorbed from the diet, so that a balance is maintained.

A woman is at a disadvantage. Like a man she loses iron each day in shed cells, but she loses additional amounts as well. Women menstruate, and menstrual blood contains, on average, about 30 mg of iron, which is equivalent to a daily loss of 1 mg. Moreover, when a woman becomes pregnant she requires more iron. Some of this, as I have mentioned, is given to her foetus, and more is needed because a pregnant woman makes a larger volume of blood in her body than when she was not pregnant and some of this is lost during childbirth. Altogether, pregnancy makes an additional demand of about 500 mg (or about $\frac{1}{50}$ oz) of iron.

In the body iron, like calcium, is dynamic. The red blood cells, like all other living things, have their own life cycle. They are made, they live, they age, and they die. A red blood cell has a life of about 120 days so that on any one day $\frac{1}{120}$ of the 250,000 million of your red blood cells die. Put another way, each day 2,000 million red blood cells die in your body. These dead red blood cells release about 27 mg of iron which becomes available for the 2,000 million new red blood cells which are formed each day in your bone marrow. Extra iron is needed to compensate for the loss of iron in the shed skin and gut cells, and in women to replace the iron lost in menstrual blood. And of course, if you lose blood in an accident, or because you have bleeding haemorrhoids or a bleeding duodenal ulcer, you will need additional iron. In the tropics extra iron is needed if you happen to have hookworms which are very common there. Hookworms fasten on to the gut wall, like leeches fasten on to the skin, and suck blood. It is quite remarkable how much blood is lost as a result of a heavy hookworm infestation. In a study made in Malaya it was found that 30 ml (1 oz) of blood was lost each day if the person had a moderate infestation (500 worms), but it rose to 80 ml (or 3 oz) a day in heavy infestations of over 1,000 worms.

In Western nations, people who take analgesics such as aspirin regularly to give them a 'lift' or to prevent headaches not only risk damaging their kidneys, but also lose some extra blood, because the analgesic irritates the stomach and slight bleeding occurs.

The iron needed to replace that lost to the body is obtained from food, and the best iron-containing foods are meat, eggs, some vegetables, and cereals. The meat need not be red meat. In fact, chicken contains as much iron as beef, and eggs contain about the same amount (2.5–3.5 mg per 100 g). Cereals such as wheat contain nearly twice as much iron per 100 g as meat, but cereals also contain phytate, which prevents iron being absorbed, so they are less useful suppliers of iron. In fact, in most Western industrialized nations, bread is 'fortified' with additional iron.

Unfortunately, only 5–25 per cent of iron in the food is absorbed, the rest is lost in the faeces. The amount absorbed depends on the sex of the person, the type of diet eaten, and whether he or she is anaemic or not. A man eating a typical Western diet (which provides more than 25 per cent of the calories from animal protein) absorbs between 6 and 10 per cent of the iron in the diet, and a woman eating a similar diet will absorb about 14 per cent of the iron. If she is pregnant she absorbs about 20 per cent. People who are anaemic absorb between 20 and 30 per cent of the iron in their food.

In contrast, the vast majority of people in the world eat a diet consisting mainly of cereals, in which animal foods provide 10 per cent or less of the calories. A person eating this kind of diet will absorb far less iron, because most of it is bound to the phytate in the cereal. Five per cent of the iron in wheat is absorbed, about 3 per cent of the iron in maize is absorbed, but only 1 per cent of the iron in rice gets into the body.

It is small wonder that iron deficiency nutritional anaemia is so widespread. And it is.

Anaemia, and the use of iron to treat it, has been known for over 2,000 years. The ancient Hindus prepared a mixture which was called Laula Bhasma by roasting sheets of iron and then pounding them into a fine powder. The powder was mixed in oil, or whey, or milk, and was given to cure pallor and weakness. The Greek doctors believed that iron, which was the metal of Ares, the god of war, would give strength to the weak. And the Roman physicians used to allow old swords to rust in tubs of water, bottles of which were then given to patients who complained of weakness or pallor.

But it took nearly 2,000 years before an English physician, Dr Sydenham, recognized that iron cured anaemia, which in those days was called chlorosis, or the 'green disease'. It particularly affected young women. In 1681, Sydenham wrote, 'I comfort the blood and the spirit belonging to it by giving a chalybeate* 30 days running. This is sure to do good. To the worn-out or languid blood it gives a spur or fillip whereby the animal spirits which before lay prostrate and sunken under their own weight are raised and excited. Clear proof of this is found in the effect of steel in chlorosis. The pulse gains strength, the face (no longer pale and deathlike) a fresh ruddy colour.'

Today among the poor, especially in the hungry developing nations, anaemia is common, although not many young Western women suffer from chlorosis. In some cases anaemia has been aggravated by civilization. When all cooking was done in iron pots, a considerable amount of the iron from the pot was eaten with the food. Increasingly, the iron cooking pot is being replaced by aluminium cooking pots, and this source of iron has been lost. The value of the iron cooking pot in preventing anaemia can be judged from the rarity of anaemia amongst the Bantu in rural South Africa. The Bantu cook their maize in iron cooking pots, and in addition drink Kaffir beer. A South African scientist, Dr Bothwell, measured the iron content in the livers of 147 Africans who had died in accidents. In 131 of them the amount exceeded the maximum he expected to find and was far more than the amount found in the livers of Europeans. The Bantu men were certainly not anaemic, and yet from their diet you would have expected them to be anaemic. Dr Bothwell attributed this to the use of iron cooking pots for food and to the habit of drinking beer, which contains a fair amount of iron.

When you go to a doctor or a laboratory to find out if you are anaemic, he usually takes a sample of blood and measures the amount of haemoglobin in it on a small machine. The result tells him the concentration of haemoglobin in a certain amount of blood and since the normal level is known, a low concentration indicates that the person has anaemia.

Anaemia is only the tip of the iceberg of nutritional iron deficiency. Before the blood shows anaemia, all the stores of iron in the body will have given up their supply to try and keep up the blood level within the normal range. Once anaemia is diag-

---

* A chalybeate was a mixture of iron filings steeped in cold wine.

nosed, the stores are empty, and the person is truly deficient in iron. To be quite sure that this is so the doctor usually does further tests on the blood, but the haemoglobin estimation is so easy to perform that a large number of people in a community can be screened to see how common anaemia is.

Investigations made in Britain, Sweden, Norway, and Germany have shown that while about 3 per cent of men were anaemic, between 5 and 25 per cent of women chosen from the community at random were anaemic.

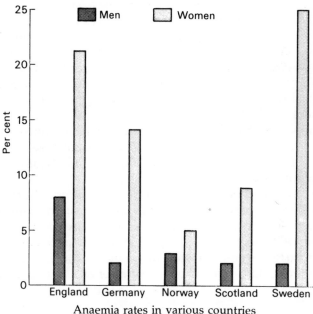

Anaemia rates in various countries

The degree of anaemia was usually quite mild, and few, if any, of the women had any symptoms; in fact they all felt perfectly healthy. However, the importance of the surveys demonstrates that women, because of menstruation, pregnancy, and lactation, rapidly empty their iron stores and so are vulnerable to anaemia unless they obtain sufficient iron in their diets, or take iron tablets.

In the affluent Western nations it is quite surprising that this can occur. Most Western diets contain between 60 and 90 g of protein, and most protein-rich foods also contain iron. This sort of diet should provide all the iron needed. Women need more iron than men, but even then a woman's average daily iron loss is only 2 mg. This amount is replaced if 11 mg of iron is available in the diet (as 20 per cent is absorbed from food).

Yet anaemia in women still seems to occur. This caused scientists to ask if the diet eaten by many women was providing the necessary quantity of iron. In the U.S.A. Dr White found the average amount of iron provided in the diet eaten by many girls and women ranged from 8 to 14 mg a day. Surprisingly, amongst university students he found the average dietary iron eaten was only 8.5 mg a day. In another investigation of women university students, Dr Monson and his associates found an average daily intake of 9.2 mg of iron. Across the Atlantic, in Göteborg, Sweden, Professor Hallberg reported that an average 15-year-old girl obtained about 11.5 mg of dietary iron a day, and that this decreased to 8.5 mg a day in the diet of elderly women.

It appeared that although iron-rich protein and cereal foods were available, many women in affluent nations were eating diets high in sugar and taking snacks of 'junk' foods rather than eating nutritious foods.

The combined factors of a lack of dietary iron, and the change from iron to aluminium or glass cooking pots has severely reduced the iron available among women in two of the richest nations of the world. Over the years this has depleted their iron stores, so that eventually when the women become pregnant or reach their mid-thirties, the symptoms of anaemia appear.

If this is the situation in the rich, industrialized nations in the West, what happens in the poor nations of the developing world? In these countries only about 10 per cent of the daily calories comes from animal foods, and nearly 80 per cent comes from cereals, usually rice, maize, and wheat, which have a low iron content and contain phytate which prevents the available iron from being absorbed. The answer to the question is therefore obvious. Large numbers of men and women, and particularly large numbers of pregnant women, are severely anaemic.

This is a serious matter. In an investigation in Malaysia, my colleagues and I found that women who were anaemic in pregnancy were five times as likely to die during pregnancy or childbirth, and were six times as likely to have a still-born baby or a baby which died in the first weeks of life, compared with non-anaemic women. (There is also some grave concern among paediatricians that babies of mothers who were anaemic during pregnancy may have diminished mental ability because their brains received insufficient oxygen during a crucial period of brain growth.) Other medical scientists in other countries of the developing world have found a similar, or worse situation.

The World Health Organization believes that anaemia affects over 40 per cent of women in the developing nations, if Western standards of diagnosing anaemia are accepted. Among pregnant women the prevalence of anaemia is even higher. Men are less affected and probably no more than 10 per cent of them are anaemic.

This means that more than 500 million people in the world are anaemic. Admittedly most of them show no signs of anaemia. They are not particularly pale, or weak, or short of breath. They manage to do a day's work. This is because their bodies have adjusted to the lower level of haemoglobin in their blood. But when a stress situation occurs, such as pregnancy, infection, or an accident, they are less well able to withstand it and become much more seriously ill, or may even die. Anaemia is considered by most experts to be partly responsible for the high mortality rates from disease and childbirth found in the developing nations.

This harm to human life could be eliminated easily and cheaply by making iron available. It can be done in two ways. The first way is to fortify foods with iron. In several industrialized nations, bread is fortified by law, with small amounts of iron added to the flour. Unfortunately, the value of this method of providing the needed iron is doubtful. English medical scientists led by Dr Elwood carried out some very sophisticated investigations into the value of fortified bread. After two years' work, they came to the conclusion that the iron was very poorly absorbed from a normal diet, and if too much iron was added, the flour became rancid quickly. Another investigation in Latin America by Dr Layrisse and his colleagues came to the same unhappy conclusion. Using iron 'tagged' with isotopes and incorporated into various foods, or given as a supplement, they found an adequate amount of iron would only be absorbed from food if animal protein was eaten as part of the daily diet. Unfortunately, the very people who need the extra iron are those who cannot afford to eat meat except on rare feast days.

But research into fortifying food with iron must and will continue. We will need to know which form of iron, usually a salt, is the most suitable. We will have to know which are the most suitable foodstuffs to be fortified with iron. We will have to know the amounts of the suitable foods which are eaten by different groups of the population. We will have to know how much of the iron added to the food is absorbed into the person's body from his gut. We will have to be sure that the consumer, and the food industry, accepts the fortified food. We will need to find out if any additional substances, such as vitamin C, for example, will enhance iron absorption.

This is urgently needed research, of far greater value in practical terms than finding a cure for cancer or methods of safely transplanting human hearts. But unfortunately because of national prestige and a distorted system of values, it has had a low priority to date.

The second way to eliminate iron-deficiency anaemia is to pay attention to hygiene: to eliminate, as far as possible, the menace of hookworm, and in Africa, bilharziasis; and to provide iron tablets to those people who are at the greatest risk of becoming anaemic. If every woman (except in the high income group) in the industrialized nations took an iron pill on the days she was not taking The Pill and if every pregnant woman took at least one iron tablet every day throughout her pregnancy, anaemia would be largely eliminated, at least until old age.

Anaemia is one of the most common diseases in the world. It could be eliminated very cheaply with an immense improvement in the health, well-being, and energy of many people, especially women.

It would be of still more value to human happiness if the rich nations were to give supplies of iron tablets to the poor nations, so that every woman was able to receive the amount of iron she needed. But for this to succeed, an educational campaign would

be needed using the radio and the press, and even more important, 'barefoot' doctors would need to be trained to be available
in the villages and to 'sell' to the people the need to take iron.

Anaemia is too important a disease to be left in the hands of
the medical profession!

As in most nutritional matters, the lack of one needed mineral or
vitamin is often found in association with other deficiencies.
Iron is no exception. People whose diet provides insufficient
iron frequently eat a diet which provides insufficient protein,
and certainly insufficient animal protein. The more meat there is
in the diet the better the iron found in other foods is absorbed.
People on a poor diet often eat insufficient vitamin C. This
applies to the poor of all ages in the hungry developing nations,
and in the rich developed nations to the ill, the old, and to those
workers on the lowest wages. If the diet does not contain a
reasonable amount of vitamin C, anaemia may result as the iron
in foods is less readily absorbed. The poorer the diet, the more
cereal it is likely to contain, and the less iron is likely to be
absorbed, because of phytate.

And it doesn't stop there. In the bone marrow red blood cells
are constantly being formed. As they develop they go through a
series of changes in shape and size until they are fully mature
and are released into the blood-stream to carry out their
evolutionary ordained function of transporting oxygen from the
lungs to the tissues of the body. The maturing process takes
about 10 days to complete and, at a precise time during the
growing period, iron is absorbed into the red cells to form the
complex oxygen-carrying substance, haemoglobin. As the red
cell matures it becomes smaller and a more efficient oxygen
transporter, but it can only achieve maturity if two vitamins are
available. These are vitamin B_{12} and folic acid. A lack of the
vitamins prevents the cell from becoming fully mature so that an
inefficient, immature cell is let out into the circulation, and
because the process is slowed down, fewer cells are let out, so
that the person eventually shows signs of anaemia. This
anaemia is called megaloblastic anaemia because many of
the red blood cells are big (megalo) and immature (blastic)
cells.

Folic acid-deficiency anaemia is the most common megalo-blastic anaemia, and it is due to a lack of green leafy vegetables in the diet. The vitamin was first found in spinach leaves in 1941, hence the name folic—from the Latin word for a leaf, *folium*.

However, the vitamin is found in other leafy vegetables and in liver, kidney, mushrooms, and yeast. In fact it was the discovery that certain women had severe anaemia in pregnancy that led scientists to suspect the presence of the vitamin.

In 1931 Lucy Wills was working amongst poor Hindu women in Calcutta. She noticed that some pregnant women had a severe anaemia which did not respond to iron treatment. The women were very pale and lethargic and often had swollen legs. Dr Wills reported that they looked as if they had pernicious anaemia but without the nervous signs found in that disease. As well as this, the anaemia did not respond to the refined liver extract injections which were being used with success to treat pernicious anaemia, but it did respond to injections of crude liver, or a diet of raw liver. Because, in some ways, the condition resembled beri-beri, Lucy Wills gave some of her patients yeast extract, which was available as marmite, and iron tablets. To her delight the anaemia was cured; in fact the marmite worked even better than the crude liver injections she had been giving. She wrote a report which was published in the *British Medical Journal*. In this she speculated that the anaemia was due to a deficiency of an unknown substance which she believed was a member of the vitamin B group.

She was right that the anaemia was due to a vitamin deficiency but she was wrong in thinking it was a B vitamin deficiency.

It took over 12 years to discover what the vitamin was. In 1943, scientists working in England and in the U.S.A. isolated the vitamin from crude liver extracts. Oddly when its chemical structure was worked out it was discovered that it was chemically related to a pigment found in butterfly wings. This gives it its chemical name, pteroylglutamic acid. The human body cannot manufacture folic acid and man has to obtain it from meat, offal, or leafy vegetables, but if these are overcooked, much of the folic acid is destroyed. Normally man needs only a tiny amount of folic acid each day, so that he generally gets enough to prevent megaloblastic anaemia. But in pregnancy, women need two or three times as much folic acid, because the vitamin is needed by the growing foetus. And if women do not eat a diet which includes green leafy vegetables, or are not given supplements of folic acid, megaloblastic anaemia may develop with apparent astonishing rapidity. In the affluent nations, folic acid-deficiency anaemia affects fewer than 1 in every 100 pregnant women, mostly the poorest. But in the hungry developing nations megaloblastic anaemia affects over 5 per cent of pregnant women, and is a hazard to their well-being and to their life.

Vitamin B_{12} is also essential for the proper development of the red blood cells, but it was only discovered 30 years ago.

Nearly 100 years before that discovery, a physician at Guy's Hospital in London, Thomas Addison, had observed that certain anaemic patients did not respond to iron therapy, but slowly became weaker and weaker, with increasing difficulty in walking, until death eventually occurred after a few years. As Dr Addison could not find a cure for the anaemia, and as it inexorably, perniciously, led to death, he called the disease pernicious anaemia.

For over 120 years, the victims of pernicious anaemia continued to go their slow, painful way to the grave. Then, in 1921, Dr Minot, who was Professor of Medicine at Harvard University in the U.S.A., reported that pernicious anaemia could be relieved if the victim ate at least a pound of raw liver each day. It was a desperate cure for a desperate disease. But it did offer hope of survival to the patient, and it gained a Nobel Prize for Dr Minot. The biochemists began to work and soon the huge quantities of liver were replaced by liver injections. But the reason why liver was so effective eluded medical scientists until the 1940s, when two groups, one in Britain and the other in the U.S.A., isolated 20 mg of the active substance from a ton of raw liver. A person needs only a thousandth part of a milligram of the crystalline vitamin to prevent pernicious anaemia. As the vitamin is found in liver, in meat, and in dairy products, which most people include in their diet, the disease is uncommon, unless you choose your parents unwisely. Unfortunately, people who develop pernicious anaemia have a defect which prevents them from transporting the tiny amount of vitamin B_{12} they need through the wall of their gut. Without the vitamin,

Every body

the red blood cells cannot mature properly and anaemia results. As well as this the vitamin is needed by nerves, and when it is lacking, various unpleasant nerve disorders result. Today, once pernicious anaemia has been diagnosed it can be treated by injections of a synthetic vitamin B_{12} produced in the laboratory.

6

An A, D, E, B, C of vitamins

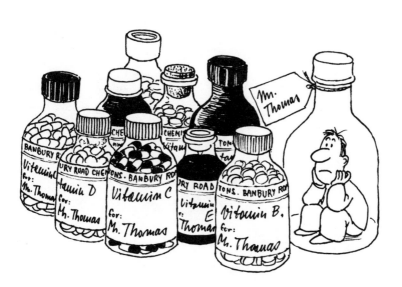

'Probably no single class of drugs has been the target of as much quackery, misunderstanding, misrepresentation, and misuse as the vitamins, despite the fact that far more is known about these compounds, including their mechanism of action, than about any other group of substances in the United States Pharmacopoea.'   *Paul Greengard, Professor of Pharmacology,*
Yale University School of Medicine.

Everyone knows about vitamins. Unless enough of them are provided in your diet you are likely to become ill because of vitamin deficiency. What is less well known is that if you ingest too much of certain vitamins you can become ill.

Technically, vitamins are organic compounds which are involved in enzyme systems in the body and have to be supplied in the diet, because the body has lost the ability to make them. They were unknown until about 70 years ago, although some perceptive nutritional scientists were beginning to realize that food consisted of more than carbohydrates, fats, and protein, and that other factors in the diet might be responsible for protection against disease.

In 1912 a famous experiment was carried out by Frederick Gowland Hopkins in Cambridge University. In an attempt to discover the effects of diet on the growth of young rats, he fed one group of rats on a special diet consisting of protein, fats, and carbohydrates, together with minerals. The second group were given the same diet, but, in addition, each rat was given about a teaspoonful of milk each day. The rats given the special diet failed to grow, but those which received the diet with the milk supplement thrived and developed normally. After 18 days, Professor Hopkins withdrew the milk from the second group of rats and gave it to the first group. The results were the reverse of the first part of the experiment. The rats which previously had been deprived of milk now began to grow normally, while the rats which previously had had milk, but were now deprived of it, ceased to grow. Hopkins argued that milk contained an 'accessory factor' essential for growth. Because of his interest in proteins, which are made up of 'building blocks' of 20 amino-acids, he believed that the accessory factor was an amino-acid or an amine. Hopkins' paper was read by a Polish biochemist, Dr Funk, who called the new substances 'vitamines' because he thought that all the accessory factors were 'vital' amines. It is now known that most are not, but the name without the final 'e' has stuck.

Further research in several laboratories quickly identified other vital amines which, as they were discovered, were given a letter and called vitamins A, B, C, D, E. In the past 50 years, most of the vitamins have been identified chemically and given new chemical names, but the old alphabetical list persists, and is convenient.

The research has shown that the vitamins can be divided into two main groups; those that are soluble in fat and those that are soluble in water. The human body is unable to maintain a large store of the water-soluble vitamins B and C, so that deficiency disease is likely to arise after a few weeks or months if the diet is deficient in these vitamins. In contrast, the human liver stores the fat-soluble vitamins A, D, and E, so a well-fed adult has sufficient stores to protect him for months should the diet contain insufficient fat-soluble vitamins.

In the case of infants and young children the situation is different. Unless an expectant mother eats a diet rich in vitamins A and D, and continues to eat it during the time she breast-feeds, the child will be unable to build up adequate stores of the vitamins in its liver.

Once the child is weaned it must obtain foods containing vitamins or it is likely to become vitamin deficient quite quickly, particularly as vitamin requirements are high under the age of 5 when body growth is rapid.

A little night-blindness

In the Second World War the story was put out that the night fighter pilots were being given additional rations of carrots (which contain vitamin A) so that they would see the enemy bombers better. The explanation was false, but it is true that deficiency in vitamin A leads to difficulty in vision when the light is dim.

Perhaps more important, at least to the millions of children in the hungry developing world, is the fact that vitamin A is necessary for growth of bone and for the normal growth and shedding of surface tissues. Every day the outermost cells of the skin, the gut, and the cornea of the eye die and are shed like leaves perpetually falling from a tree. But unlike the leaves on a tree, new cells immediately replace them. The process of shedding only proceeds normally if there is sufficient vitamin A circulating in the blood and seeping into the tissues. In the absence of an adequate supply, the surface tissues, particularly of the eyes, fail to shed the dead cells. These then collect on the surface so that it becomes dry and thickened. In the eyes a hazy opaque film across the cornea develops, and if it is not treated promptly by giving vitamin A, the cornea may soften and collapse, causing blindness.

Each year tens of thousands of children in the developing nations become permanently blind because of the lack of minute amounts of vitamin A in their daily food. Vitamin A is found mainly in butter, cheese, and milk and in liver and fish-liver oils. The body is also able to make it from carotene, the yellow pigment found in many fruits and vegetables. But in most tropical countries dairy foods are expensive, fish-liver oils and liver not eaten, and because of food taboos children can only eat certain fruits. In these areas too diarrhoeal diseases are common so that less of the scarce vitamin A is absorbed at a time when more is needed.

The blindness due to vitamin A deficiency is rare in prosperous communities, but is still a cause of misery and despair in many developing nations. It has been calculated that in some areas, one in every hundred children under the age of 5 becomes blind as a result of vitamin A deficiency. This blindness is entirely preventable. If all the children were given supplements of vitamin A from birth, and if mothers learnt about nutrition at school and in community centres, it would cease to be a problem. Vitamin A, or retinol, is cheap, and if sugar or salt used by the people in the affected parts of the developing world were 'fortified' with vitamin A, the blindness would disappear. It would cost no more than U.S. 15 c. a head a year to eliminate this misery. To obtain the same amount of vitamin A needed from vegetable or fruit it would be necessary to eat three times as much of the former and twice as much of the latter.

If you live in the rich, developed nations of the world you are unlikely to need vitamin A supplements, unless you belong to a poverty-stricken deprived minority. You certainly should avoid taking large doses of vitamin A in 'high-dose capsules', since they may cause liver damage.

The case of the twisted bones

The industrial revolution of the nineteenth century in north-
west Europe led to a drift of people from the rural areas to the
new towns which had sprung up around the factories. As the
revolution gathered momentum, the drift increased and the
'dark satanic mills', so graphically named by William Blake,
were surrounded by small back-to-back workmen's cottages.
The factories belched out smoke to cloud the sky so that even in
summer the towns lay under the shroud of industrial pollution.
Charles Dickens, writing in 1854, described one of these industrial towns in his book *Hard Times*, calling it Coketown. He
wrote:

> It was a town of red brick, or of brick that would have been red if
> the smoke and ashes had allowed it; but, as matters stood it was a
> town of unnatural red and black like the painted face of a savage. It
> was a town of machinery and tall chimneys, out of which inter-
> minable serpents of smoke trailed themselves for ever and ever,
> and never got uncoiled. . . .

Even in midsummer the sun in Coketown was hidden. . . .

> Seen from a distance in such weather, Coketown lay shrouded in a
> haze of its own, which appeared impervious to the sun's rays. You
> only knew the town was there, because you knew there could have
> been no such sulky blotch upon the prospect without a town. . . .

And within the town, the conditions were ideal for diseases to
afflict the children of the workers. . . .

> In the hardest working part of Coketown, in the innermost fortifi-
> cations of that ugly citadel where Nature was so strongly bricked
> out as killing airs and gases were bricked in; at the heart of the
> labyrinth of narrow courts upon courts and close streets upon
> streets . . . were built in an immense variety of stunted and
> crooked shapes as though every house put out a sign of the kind of
> people who might be expected to be born in it; lived the people.

The hours of work were long, the pay poor, the threat of
dismissal great. Food was indeed more plentiful than in rural
areas, but what was gained in quantity was lost in quality.

It is not surprising that children growing up in this environment were poorly fed. They ate a diet mainly composed of bread
and dripping, with occasional meat meals. They lived in the

squalid narrow streets from which the sun was excluded by the smoke and dust pouring up from the factories. In 1884 a survey of the distribution of rickets in Britain showed that the disease was common in industrial towns, and uncommon in the country. On Clydeside every child examined was found to be affected. Six years later a survey by Dr Thomas Palin showed that the disease was common where sunshine was scarce, and rare where sunshine was abundant. This was a new and unwelcome concept. Eminent physicians who had formed their own, often exclusive, theories were not going to accept such a simple suggestion. The disease must be due to infection, or a disturbance of a gland, or to lack of exercise, they said. With tenacious persistence, each clung to his favourite theory and refused to be shifted, although over the years two theories gained increasing support. These were that rickets was either due to deprivation of sunshine, as Dr Palin had suggested, or it was caused by a defective diet. The latter theory became increasingly popular after Professor Hopkins had written in 1906, 'In diseases such as rickets, and particularly in scurvy, we have had for long years knowledge of a dietetic factor'; and Dr Funk had written in 1914, 'It is very probable that rickets occurs only when certain substances in the diet essential for normal metabolism are lacking or are supplied in insufficient amount. The substances occur in good breast milk, also in cod-liver oil.'

This remark may have stimulated Edward Mellanby in London to experiment by giving puppies various diets to see if rickets developed. Puppies were known to be particularly susceptible to rickets. Mellanby approached the problem scientifically. He established a standard diet which regularly produced rickets in puppies, and then added different food substances, in turn, to see if rickets was prevented. After nearly 400 experiments he was able to report in 1921 that cod-liver oil and, to a lesser extent, peanut oil and butter contained some substance which protected the puppies against rickets. He failed to notice that if the puppies were kept out of doors, rickets was less likely to develop, but he did remark that confinement of the puppies in cages contributed to the development of the disease.

Surprisingly, the suggestion by Dr Funk and Professor Mellanby that cod-liver oil protected against rickets was not new. Folk medicine among people living on the coasts of England,

Holland, and France, had recommended cod-liver oil as a specific for rickets for generations! And amongst the peasants, rickets was never found. In 1921 two American scientists, Drs Shipley and Park, discovered how cod-liver oil prevents rickets. They argued that rickets was caused either by a lack of sunshine, or by a diet which was deficient in an unknown substance, which they called X. X was found in fish-liver oils, and was present in butter, but butter fat contained very little compared with cod-liver oil. Quite soon it was discovered that substance X was a fat-soluble vitamin, which was named vitamin D. Vitamin D, or calciferol, was found in large quantities in cod-liver oil (and in other fish-liver oils).

But why should sunlight also prevent rickets? The answer to that problem was also quickly found. Sunlight, by irradiating the skin, caused the body to convert an inert substance in the skin called 7-dehydrocholesterol, into vitamin D. In the industrial cities the smoke pall which filled the sky prevented the ultraviolet rays of the sun from penetrating into the streets, and the children rarely, if ever, ate fish-liver oils. The deficiency of calciferol prevented calcium in the diet from being absorbed, mobilized, and deposited in the bones, so that the bones became softer than normal. In infancy and childhood bone growth is rapid, and with a lack of the normal mineralization of bone, the bones softened and became twisted. Rickets developed. This occurred especially when the child began to walk, because the weight of the body on the softened bones led to bowed legs and arms, and to knock-knees. The shape of the pelvis became distorted, thus (if the child was a girl) making childbearing difficult in later life.

Once the cause of the disease had been found, a reasonable person would assume that it would have been eliminated at once. Cod-liver oil is cheap. Yet a survey made of infants in 1943 showed that in Leeds, Newcastle, and Manchester, 4 per cent of the children had rickets. In Dublin and Belfast 9 per cent, and in Sheffield, 10 per cent of the infants examined had the disease.

This led to a campaign to eliminate the disease in areas where the hours of sunshine are few and industrial smog considerable. In Britain, with wartime food rationing in operation, pregnant women and young children were given vitamin D capsules and mothers were advised to put their infants out in the sun when it shone. This has led to the virtual disappearance of rickets in Britain, but recently it has begun to appear again as coloured immigrant children leave the sunny tropics and go to live in the cloudy nations of Europe and North America. There is some evidence that a dark pigmented skin may impede the passage of ultraviolet rays, and the reduction of the hours of exposure to sunshine in temperate countries may be sufficient to precipitate mild rickets. Rickets also persists in some tropical developing countries where children are wrapped and kept indoors, rather than being allowed to play freely in the abundant sunshine. Some adult women in Asian countries who are kept in purdah develop vitamin D deficiency and softened bones because they are never exposed to sunlight and their diet is deficient in vitamin D. In adult life the disease is called osteomalacia. Osteomalacia may also affect elderly people (particularly solitary men) living on restricted diets in the developed nations. But it is very uncommon.

In all cases of disease due to vitamin D deficiency, the cure is simple. It is to supply a diet rich in calcium and phosphorus and to give an appropriate dose of vitamin D each day.

Today, in most countries, young children are exposed to the sun judiciously; and in countries with a low number of hours of sunshine, cow's milk fortified with vitamin D is available. In addition, infants and very young children are usually given daily vitamin D supplements. Old people would also be wise to take vitamin D supplements, particularly if they eat a restricted diet. But perhaps a seat in a sunny corner with a gossiping friend might be an even better way of preventing vitamin D deficiency.

Excessive ingestion of vitamin D, in the false belief that if a little vitamin does you some good, a lot will do you far more good, can be dangerous. If too much vitamin D is given to babies, they lose their appetite, and become irritable and depressed. The excessive amounts of vitamin causes a much greater than normal absorption of calcium from the milk the baby drinks, and paradoxically removes calcium from parts of its bones, causing a disease. But this is not usual, and most people affected by excessive vitamin D intake are adults who have read somewhere that large doses of the vitamin benefit certain diseases, notably rheumatoid arthritis. There is no evidence that the vitamin *does* help, but people are gullible. The individual who develops vitamin D toxicity becomes weak and has headaches, tiredness, and bouts of vomiting and diarrhoea. Later his kidneys may be affected, and if the excessive amounts are eaten over a long period, his blood vessels may become calcified. Excessive vitamin D can be harmful in another way. It raises the level of the cholesterol in the blood, and as is shown in Chapter 8, this may be a cause of coronary heart disease. Recently Professor Linden, who practises in Tromso in northern Norway, has reported that some people with heart disease had taken significantly larger amounts of vitamin D over the years than randomly selected people of the same age and sex who had no heart disease.

The amount of vitamin D required to cause toxicity varies, but the condition will not occur if the daily intake is less than 50 micrograms, and usually ten times that amount has to be taken each day. The average daily needs of vitamin D for infants and children under the age of 5 is 10 micrograms, which is also the requirement for pregnant and lactating women. All other people, of both sexes and of all ages, require no more than 2.5 micrograms a day. Since butter and margarine contain vitamin D, most people obtain all the vitamin D they need from the food they eat and supplements are unnecessary. In some countries milk is fortified with vitamin D so that vitamin capsules are not strictly necessary provided children play in the sun.

E—A vitamin in search of a disease

In 1922 a group of research scientists in the University of California fed a colony of rats on a special diet which contained all the nutrients known to be essential at that time. The rats thrived on this diet, but the females failed to reproduce normally, and almost all their foetuses died before birth. When fresh lettuce, yeast, wheat, oats, dried alfalfa, meat, and milk were added to their diet, the females reproduced normal offspring. The inference obviously was that the special diet lacked an essential nutrient, probably a vitamin. Eventually this missing vitamin was identified as a fat-soluble alcohol, and was named tocopherol from the Greek words, *tocos* meaning childbirth, and *phero* meaning to bring forth or deliver. The alternative name, adopted by nutritional scientists obsessed with sequential classification, was vitamin E, for this was the letter available for the vitamin which was discovered next. By 1938, vitamin E, or alpha-tocopherol, had been synthesized in the laboratory and research began in earnest. Diets containing various quantities of vitamin E, or no vitamin E at all, were fed to rats, rabbits, chickens, dogs, sheep, and cattle to find out what happened. The results were bizarre and varied quite considerably, depending on the species investigated. For example, if male rats were fed diets deficient in vitamin E, the sperm-producing cells in their testicles degenerated, as did their livers. Chickens developed brain damage, muscular inco-ordination and eventually paralysis, and calves developed heart disease.

It was argued that if a deficiency of vitamin E caused these serious conditions in animals, a lack of vitamin E might also be the cause of impotence and sterility in men, repeated abortions in women, muscular weakness in both sexes, and might be a cause of coronary heart disease. But over the years, in a wide variety of clinical situations, no human given extra vitamin E showed any improvement. It remained a 'vitamin in search of a disease'. One reason was that vitamin E is normally found in many foodstuffs eaten by man. It is not destroyed by cooking, and the normal diet provides for more than the recommended daily requirements of 5–30 mg. Since vitamin E acts as an antioxidant, preventing fats in the body from being broken down by oxygen, the higher intake is needed by people who eat large quantities of fats. It was also discovered that people who ate polyunsaturated fats in preference to saturated fats needed more vitamin E, as polyunsaturated fats are more likely to be oxidized. This led to the suggestion that people who had heart attacks and had been induced to eat margarine rather than butter, and fish in preference to beef, should have vitamin E supplements. The argument was only half true. The fact that polyunsaturated fat eaters needed a larger daily intake to prevent fat oxidization was true, but since margarine (which is made from polyunsaturated fats) contains nearly 15 times as much vitamin E as butter, and fish 10 times as much as red meat, additional vitamin E supplements are unnecessary.

In order to see if a deficiency of vitamin E harmed man, Dr Howitt, head of the Biochemical Research Laboratories at the

Elgin State Hospital in Illinois, was given a commission in 1967 by the U.S. National Research Council to find out what happened to people given a diet containing only one-third the amount of vitamin E found in a typical American diet. The results showed that the low-vitamin E subjects were as healthy and as active in every way as people eating ordinary diets, despite the reduction of their blood plasma alpha-tocopherol by 80 per cent. The only abnormality found was that their red blood cells only lived for 110 days instead of living an average of 120 days. Dr Howitt concluded that humans need only a modest amount of vitamin E and this amount is provided in the diet even if it is a poor one. He admitted that in exceptional circumstances a deficiency in vitamin E might lead to disease, but it was most unlikely to occur.

In 1967 it did—in exceptional circumstances. In one hospital in the United States premature babies were fed on a synthetic milk substitute because it was believed they would thrive better than if they were given human milk or cow's milk. The mixture contained a higher proportion of protein, and a lower proportion of fat. The babies did thrive, but eleven developed a blood disease: haemolytic anaemia, in which the red blood cells live for a shorter time than usual. Investigations revealed that the milk substitute contained very small quantities of vitamin E, and when the babies were given vitamin E supplements, the anaemia was cured. The error was in trying to be clever and giving the babies a milk substitute instead of milk. Babies with the rare congenital disease called cystic fibrosis require extra tocopherol because they are unable to absorb the quantity provided by milk feeds, but for normal babies, human milk and cow's milk contain all the vitamin E a baby requires.

For people on normal diets, vitamin E supplements are unnecessary, despite exaggerated claims which appear at intervals that the vitamin improves sexual potency and cures diseases as widely separated as recurrent abortion in women, sterility in men, coeliac disease in children, and diabetes in both sexes. The evidence, after careful study, is that the claims that vitamin E had alleviated any of these diseases are false at best and dangerously untrue at worst.

In recent years a further claim has been made for vitamin E. This is that it is a 'thrilling breakthrough in skin care', removing wrinkles, blemishes, dryness, stretch marks, smell, and that it rejuvenates ageing skin, as well as healing burns and wounds more quickly. Most of the skin creams and underarm deodorants in which vitamin E is an ingredient are marketed in the United States. With the suspicion that the claims were false, Consumers Union of U.S. Inc. searched all the reputable journals on skin disease and they contacted leading dermatologists. In no British or American dermatological journal did they find a single article, report, or letter about vitamin E in the treatment of skin diseases; and not a single dermatologist reported that he found vitamin E to be a 'thrilling breakthrough in skin care'. The claims were also investigated by the New York State's Consumer Frauds and Protection Bureau, who enquired especially from the American Medical Association's Committee on Cutaneous Health and Cosmetics. 'To date', reported the chairman in reply, 'there is absolutely no evidence that vitamin E applied to the skin is in any way beneficial to that organ.' As a final check in their investigation, Consumers Union telephoned several of the manufacturers. None could refer the investigators to any reported, or unreported controlled study of vitamin E's efficiency in skin disorders. The claims were spurious; the advertising, as one marketing director admitted, was 'on the outrageous side'. The same findings were made when the efficacy of vitamin E as an underarm deodorant was investigated. It had no effect.

In the case of skin creams containing vitamin E all that the credulous consumer loses is cash. In the case of the claims that vitamin E cures heart disease, it could lead heart disease sufferers to delay obtaining proper medical attention for their conditions. This could be serious.

What evidence is there that vitamin E helps heart disease sufferers?

The story started in Canada in 1946 when three doctors living in Ontario, Canada, claimed a dramatic cure of a boy who had acute rheumatic fever for the second time. The first attack had necessitated his admission to hospital for a prolonged period. The second attack was treated by Dr Shute, who did not think there was any need to put the boy into hospital, and reported,

'The only treatment I used for the boy was 200 units of alpha-tocopherol daily . . . in three days he was apparently well; on the sixth day he walked into my office.' Two hundred units is equivalent to 135 mg, or about ten times the recommended daily requirement. Dr Shute was the brother of Dr Evan Shute who had long advocated the use of vitamin E for the treatment of repeated abortions. Dr Shute's study was taken up enthusiastically by *Time* magazine which reported, 'Out of Canada last week came news of a startling discovery: a treatment for heart disease (the nation's No. 1 killer) which so far has succeeded against all common forms of the ailment . . . large concentrated doses of vitamin E . . . benefited four types of heart ailment (95 per cent of the total): arteriosclerotic, hypertensive, rheumatic, old and new coronary disease. The vitamin helps a failing heart. It eliminates anginal pain. It is non-toxic.'

Here was hope for millions of heart sufferers! The enthusiasm was enormous and was increased when the Shute brothers and their colleague, Dr Vogelsang, reported in 1947 that the majority of a further 84 patients who had angina pectoris—a chest pain which radiates down the left arm and is thought to be associated with coronary heart disease—had responded to vitamin E treatment.

A major problem of the Shutes' trial was that it was uncontrolled. There were no safeguards to find out if the results were really due to the treatment and not to other factors. This information is best obtained in a double-blind controlled trial: the Shute brothers used no controls, nor did they do a 'double-blind trial'. In this type of trial two groups of patients, who have been told beforehand that they are to take part in a trial of a drug, and who have volunteered to be in the trial, are matched as far as possible for numbers, age, sex, weight, and similar factors. One group is then given the actual drug being investigated, the other group a dummy. Neither the doctors attending the patients, nor the patients themselves, know who is given what until all the measurements have been made and the trial has ended. But to set up a double-blind trial is time-consuming, expensive, and complicated, so that it is usual to do initial simpler trials first. That could have excused the Shutes. By 1951, eleven trials of vitamin E as a treatment of heart disease had been reported in the medical literature. A total of 263 patients had been investigated by 26 physicians with uniformly unfavourable results.

This confirmed the 1948 report of Dr Eichart, who was also studying vitamin E and heart disease, and who wrote to the heads of departments of medicine of most of the medical schools in North America asking whether they thought vitamin E helped. The answers were uniformly that it did not. He wrote in summary, 'With the exception of the claims made by Shute and Vogelsang and their group, every published, written, or verbal report which this essayist has been able to obtain indicates that vitamin E has no value in the treatment of heart disease.' The claims made by Wilfred and Evan Shute were merely personal impressions made by men who had an infinite faith in their treatment and who had the personality to induce that faith in their patients.

Although doctors no longer use vitamin E to treat heart disease, or indeed to treat any disease, the Shute brothers and others continue to write in magazines and to publish paperback books with such titles as: *Vitamin E for Ailing and Healthy Hearts*; *Vitamin E: Your Key to a Healthy Heart*; and *Vitamin E: Key to Sexual Satisfaction*. Those who promote vitamin E capsules in health food stores and pharmacies claim that 'millions of people are currently suffering from painful, crippling, life-threatening diseases because their misguided physicians refuse to recommend vitamin E supplements to them'.

There is not an atom of truth in these claims; the advertising is deceptive, the claims are false. In a carefully worded statement issued in 1973, the National Research Council of the U.S.A. reported that a full investigation of the effects of vitamin E on human health showed them all to be false. Generously the statement reported that 'many of the claims made for vitamin E are based on misinterpretations of research on experimental animals'. For example, the statement points out that the claim for vitamin E's ability to enhance sexual potency inappropriately stems from research that showed it to be *among* the factors required to prevent sterility in male rats and to permit normal pregnancy in female rats. 'Claims that the vitamin prevents heart attacks result from a similar misinterpretation of research, says the statement. 'While a vitamin E deficiency did cause heart-muscle abnormalities in cattle and sheep, similar studies done on monkeys produced no such consequence.'

The statement further reports that the widespread distribution of vitamin E in vegetable oils, cereal grains, and animal fats makes it highly unlikely that humans ever suffer from any deficiency of the vitamin. Additional dietary supplements are therefore considered unnecessary. Vitamin E is no more a cure for anything than is snake oil or goanna juice. It remains a vitamin in search of a disease.

More than that, there is some recent concern that excessive amounts of the vitamin may cause or aggravate disease. This is of particular importance since vitamin E capsules are sold over the counter without prescription in many countries. Not only does vitamin E not protect against heart disease; it may actually increase the risk of disease developing. Both in animals and, more important, in humans, vitamin E supplements, in the dose-range of the capsules sold without prescription, increase the level of cholesterol in the blood serum. Raised serum cholesterol is thought by many medical scientists to be related to heart attacks, as I discuss in Chapter 9. In susceptible people, vitamin E supplements may cause weakness and fatigue. And perhaps more serious and sinister, if large amounts of vitamin E are eaten the vitamin may alter the breakdown of bile salts in the gut, and may—and I stress *may*—convert them into cancer-promoting substances.

For people who eat normal diets, and that is most of us, vitamin E supplements are unnecessary, and may cause or aggravate disease.

'Fresh rice is never toxic'

Until the early part of the nineteenth century most of the peoples of East Asia ate a staple diet of rice which was sown, grown, harvested, and milled in the village. Usually the milling was done laboriously in a hand mill by the women of the family. The work was hard, the husk resistant to separation from the grain.

Watt's invention of the steam engine in England and the technological advances it produced led to the introduction of power milling. The advantages were considerable. The harvested rice was taken to the mill, the husking was done mechanically, and a fine white attractive-looking rice was produced; no longer did the women have to spend hours pounding and grinding the paddy. They had more time to develop other pursuits. To the entrepreneurs of Asia, and to the European merchants, the new process was financially attractive. Engines made in the West were sold to Asia. European and Asian businessmen set up rice mills. The better the rice was milled, the more bran there was to be sold for animal food. The more rice that was milled, the more there was available for the urban dwellers, and rural labour could be diverted to other ends such as growing cotton, tea, indigo, and other cash crops, which were sold cheaply to the colonial power, and returned to the colonies as expensive manufactured goods.

Quite rapidly the mechanical methods of rice milling spread over Asia, and so did a new disease which was called beri-beri because it resembled an older disease of that name.

This disease was strange. It began with increasing fatigue, a loss of appetite, and heaviness and stiffness of the victim's legs. Labourers found that they tired easily when doing work which before had been no problem to them, and their legs became stiff and uncomfortable. Later, tingling and numb areas developed on the skin, and the calf muscles became tender so that their output of work dropped. Sleep became disturbed, with long periods of insomnia. Then, gradually, muscular weakness and wasting became apparent. The victim could no longer work. He walked supported on a stick with a swaying, staggering gait, and eventually became paralysed. In some cases his body became swollen with retained water, his breathing grew difficult as a result of fluid in his lungs. Finally his heart failed. This form of beri-beri, which was called wet beri-beri, also affected small infants aged between two and four months who died quickly.

The cause of the disease was obscure, but since it affected so many of the peasant labourers on plantations and estates, and those employed to build roads and railways to open up a country, it worried the European officials. In 1907, in the Federated Malay States, a crucial series of experiments was begun. These lasted for four years and finally uncovered the cause of beri-beri. The scientists were two young Europeans, Dr Fraser and Dr Stanton.

The first experiment was to try to find out, when other factors were excluded or controlled, if people who ate white rice would develop beri-beri and if other people under exactly the same conditions but fed on brown rice would avoid the disease. To do this it was necessary to find an isolated spot far away from any village so that infection brought in from outside could be excluded and so that the subjects involved in the experiments would be unable to buy extra food.

At that time the government was making a road in a remote· area of the state of Negri Sembilan and had recruited Javanese labourers for the job. When Dr Fraser heard about this he obtained permission to try his diets on the labourers. These men were to be the experimental group, and the experiment was to be called 'The Durian Tipus Project'. In April 1907 Fraser and Stanton travelled by train, mule, and foot to Durian Tipus and carefully examined the 300 labourers. None showed any signs of existing or previous beri-beri. The men were provided with a diet of rice, dried salt fish, onions, potatoes, coconut, tea, and salt (which was, in fact, the diet they usually ate) and were divided into two groups. The first group's rice ration was white rice. The second group were given brown rice which is steamed before picking off the husk, some of which adheres to the grain. Each group had to eat the same diet for about six months and then the groups changed over and ate the other type of rice. The rest of the rations remained identical in both groups.

The first group, eating white rice, remained well until early August. Then the first case of beri-beri appeared. A month later, four more cases had occurred, and by October a further six cases had occurred. The group were then fed brown rice and beri-beri disappeared.

The second group, eating brown rice, remained free from beri-beri for the entire six months and were changed to white rice in the middle of October. The first case of beri-beri appeared five months later and several more followed in the next month. Dr Fraser wrote, 'The general results lend support to the view that the disease beri-beri as it occurs in the Peninsula has, if not its origin, at least an intimate relation with white rice and justifies further research along these lines.'

For the next three years they continued their research. First they tried to find if white rice contained a poison, and failing to find one, thought that perhaps white rice was deficient in some protective substance. So they started to work with fowls and after many experiments found that brown rice did have a protective substance which had seeped into the rice from the outer layers of the husk during parboiling. They also found that if the 'polishings' that were left after milling the rice were added to white rice, the fowls remained healthy. It was clear to Fraser and Stanton that, as they reported in 1911, 'These researches, which comprise an unbroken sequence of experiments beginning with rices associated with outbreaks of human beri-beri demonstrated that rice is rendered harmful by the milling and polishing process to which it is subjected in the preparation of white polished rice . . . As measures for the prevention of beri-beri in this country, it is recommended that the use of unpolished, or undermilled rice be encouraged among those classes of the community in which the disease occurs.'

The same year, a research chemist called Funk was able to extract a water-soluble substance from rice-polishings that would cure beri-beri. He called it the 'beri-beri vitamin'.

By 1926 the beri-beri vitamin, called vitamin B, had been isolated in a crystalline form, and ten years later it had been made synthetically in the laboratory.

The vitamin, which is now called thiamine, is present in small amounts in all living cells and is consequently found in all natural foods. But because it is not soluble in fat it is absent from butter, animal fats, and vegetable oils. In cereals it is found in the outer layers of the grain, so that wholemeal bread is rich in the vitamin, but white flour is poor. However, in most countries thiamine is added to flour to make up the deficiency.

People in Western nations who eat a normal diet are rarely deficient in thiamine, and beri-beri is unusual. But occasionally cases occur, usually among elderly single alcoholics who exist on alcohol and little else.

For most of us, unless we are alcoholics, thiamine or vitamin B supplements are unnecessary.

Research over the past 50 years has shown that there is more than one water-soluble vitamin, but all resemble the original vitamin B in many ways. To date eight vitamins in the B complex have been isolated, although only two are associated with human deficiency diseases. The first of these is thiamine; the second is vitamin B_2 or niacin, which prevents pellagra.

Pellagra is found among maize-eating peoples. Maize, or Indian corn, was unknown in Europe until America was discovered, but there it was the staple cereal. As maize grows quickly and easily in places which are unsuitable for other cereals, it is now grown in Africa, southern Europe, and other countries.

Pellagra first appeared in Spain some time after the Spanish *conquistadores* brought back the new plant from Peru. For three centuries the cause of the disease was unknown, although in 1735 Dr Gaspar Casal of Oviedo had suggested that the new disease might be connected with eating maize. About this time a particularly severe outbreak of the disease occurred among maize eaters in Italy. The disease appeared first in spring. Exposed portions of the skin, such as the back of the hands, the forearms, and the neck, became red and itchy and small blisters appeared. The skin then hardened and became tough, blackish, and brittle. After a while the tongue became red and swollen and diarrhoea developed. In severe cases, the victim's mind became progressively clouded. The disease was called pellagra: the name comes from the Italian words *pelle* meaning skin and *agra* meaning sour. Students remember it as the disease with the three Ds: dermatitis, diarrhoea, and dementia.

Since that time thousands of mild cases of pellagra, and some hundreds of severe cases, have occurred each spring among maize-eating peasants in southern Europe, in Latin America, and the southern states of the U.S.A.

The story of the discovery of the cause of pellagra mirrors that of the discovery of the cause of beri-beri. In the early days most people refused to accept that maize was the cause. At various times pellagra was believed to be due to infection, to poison, to a disease contracted from sheep, to eating raw meat, to bad air, and to misery! The discovery that pellagra was a deficiency disease was due to the persistent work of an American, Dr Goldberger, in the deep south of the U.S.A. between 1913 and 1938. In a series of experiments he fed dogs on a maize diet and produced a condition called 'black tongue' which he claimed was similar to pellagra. In fact, when he fed the same diet to men, they developed pellagra. So he was right. He then showed that pellagra could be prevented by the addition of milk and a variety of other foods, particularly liver, kidneys, and fish, and could be cured quickly by giving yeast or yeast extracts. The fact that dogs produced similar symptoms to pellagra gave researchers a suitable laboratory animal on which to test food extracts. By 1937 the cause of pellagra had been found. It was due to the lack of a water-soluble substance of the B group called nicotinic acid or niacin. Like thiamine, niacin is found in the outer layers of wheat, so that people who eat wholemeal bread and a mixed diet are rarely deficient in the vitamin. And in many countries, including Australia, Britain, Canada, and the U.S.A., niacin must be added by law if white flour is used for bread.

Unless you are very poor and a maize-eater you don't need supplements of niacin (vitamin B_2).

The reason maize-eaters develop pellagra is because maize has only very small quantities of niacin, and also lacks an amino-acid called tryptophan which the body can convert to a limited extent into niacin. Why maize should lack this amino-acid is not known, because other cereals such as wheat, rye, rice, and barley contain tryptophan. In areas where maize is the staple cereal, and niacin-rich foods are expensive, vitamin supplements of niacin should be available, but among affluent societies supplements are not needed.

The most expensive urine in the world

In 1497 Vasco da Gama sailed from Portugal to seek a passage to the spice islands of the Orient. He sailed south along the unknown coast of Africa, and rounding the southern tip of the continent at the Cape of Good Hope he crossed the Indian Ocean to reach land on the Malabar coast of India. It was the beginning of European expansion into Asia, and the beginning of the colonial exploitation on which the economic growth of Europe was to depend.

Vasco da Gama's voyage was not without suffering. The food

on the ships was limited. Dry biscuits, decaying meat, and wine were the staple diet of the sailors. The few fruits that were taken aboard were quickly eaten. By the time the Cape was rounded, half of his crew had succumbed to a strange disease which caused swollen, sore, bleeding gums and patches of spontaneous bruising in their skins. They had developed scurvy. By the time the ship reached India, one hundred and sixty of the men had died.

Da Gama's successful and innovatory voyage opened East Asia to adventurers and merchants of Europe. The spice islands of the Indonesian archipelago held treasures that enabled Europeans to mask the dull, decayed taste of the meat they ate throughout the long northern winters. At that time it was necessary to kill the cattle in autumn, as the fodder vanished; but salt meat was dull, insipid, and often rancid. The spices hid the taste. East Asia also had silk and exotic merchandise which was desired by the rich, and merchants were prepared to risk the capital involved in mounting a speculative voyage because of the high potential profit.

Increasing numbers of ships sailed down the coast of Africa, rounded the Cape and then sailed north by east across the Indian Ocean. And on every voyage a large number of the crew became ill with scurvy, and many died. The crews were expendable, the potential profits were great, and so the voyages and the scurvy continued.

For the next three centuries sailors and others continued to die of scurvy. The disease, according to a ship's chaplain writing in 1740, caused

> large discoloured spots, dispersed upon the whole surface of the body, swelled legs, putrid gums, and above all, an extraordinary lassitude of the whole body, especially after any exercise, however inconsiderable; and this lassitude at last degenerates into a proneness to swoon, and even to die, on the least exertion of strength, or even on the least motion. This disease is likewise attended with a strange degeneration of spirits, with shiverings, tremblings, and a disposition to be seized with the most dreadful terrors on the slightest accident.

The cure, when it came, was surprisingly simple. It was to ensure that sailors were provided with fresh vegetables or, failing a supply of these, with the juice of oranges and lemons.

That was suggested in the late eighteenth century and was finally confirmed by an experiment in the British Navy. In 1796 the physician of the Channel Fleet was able to write: 'The late occurrences in the Channel Fleet have sufficiently established the fact that scurvy can always be prevented by fresh vegetables and cured effectively by the lemon or the preserved juice of that fruit . . . Whatever may be the theory of sea scurvy, we contend that recent vegetable matter imparts a *something* to the body, which fortifies it against the disease.' What the 'something' was remained obscure for over 120 years.

As the disease was apparently confined to seamen on long voyages, and was uncommon in Britain, it did not pose a problem to most doctors. The desire to find what the 'something' was, persisted in the minds of a few physicians, but little advance could be made until the accumulation of knowledge in the nineteenth century led to the development of the science of biochemistry. Even then problems remained. Clearly it was impossible to experiment with humans, and no animal apparently developed scurvy when fed a diet which would undoubtedly provoke the disease in man.

Then in 1907 guinea-pigs were found to develop the disease when placed on a diet containing no green grasses, vegetables, or fruits. Using various extracts of citrus fruit juices, which had proved so successful in preventing scurvy in sailors, scientists were able to isolate the protective factor, and it was given the name ascorbic acid because it prevented the scorbutic disease, or scurvy.

Vitamin C, or ascorbic acid, is obtained mainly from fruits and vegetables. Citrus fruits and guavas are particularly rich in the vitamin, as are some green vegetables, such as brussels sprouts and broccoli. The concentration of the vitamin in potatoes is not high, but if large amounts of potatoes are eaten, as in Ireland and Scotland, these tubers can provide most or all of the vitamin C requirements, particularly if boiled in their skins or baked. The amount of vitamin C contained in potatoes diminishes the longer they are stored, so that the previous year's crop which is eaten in late spring and early summer before the new potatoes become available may contain very little. Each year occasional cases of scurvy are diagnosed in Scotland and Ireland, usually among elderly men living alone who dislike or cannot afford to buy fresh fruits and vegetables.

The quantity of vitamin C available from vegetables and potatoes depends on the method of preparation and cooking. Vitamin C is soluble in water and is destroyed by excessive cooking. Unfortunately, the English way of cooking is to boil vegetables in large quantities of water. Not only does this reduce the original content of vitamin C by about half, but it produces a mushy, soggy end-product.

Apart from fruit and vegetables, other foods contain only small amounts of vitamin C. For example, meat, eggs, and milk contain only minute traces. Luckily the amount needed to prevent scurvy is small. It is less than 10 mg a day and at least twice that amount is contained in a single orange or other citrus fruit or in 30 ml (one oz) of fruit juice. This is exactly the daily ration recommended to the British Navy. An ordinary helping of green vegetables (about 60 g or 2 oz) if it is not boiled to mush, provides 25 mg of vitamin C, and 120 g (4 oz) of potatoes provides about the same amount, so that a normal diet will protect most people from scurvy.

To make quite sure that scurvy is prevented and to allow for individual variations in the way that food is prepared and cooked and which foods are eaten, the Nutritional Committee of the Medical Research Council in the U.K. in 1969 recommended a daily intake of 30 mg of vitamin C, and the Food and Nutritional Board in the U.S.A. in 1968 one of 60 mg. This larger amount was to allow for conditions of infection or stress when it is known extra vitamin C is needed by the body.

Most people living in the developed nations eat a diet which provides at least 30 mg of vitamin C, and often more than 60 mg of the vitamin daily, so that supplements of vitamin C are usually unnecessary, and merely pass through the body to be excreted in the urine. There are exceptions. Two researchers in Australia, Dr Joan Woodhill, who is a nutritionist, and Dr Sylvia Nobile, a chemist, found in 1973 that the risk of scurvy is quite serious among elderly people living in Sydney. They found that over three-quarters of 22 women aged 67–89 and 21 men aged 60–86 did not have their tissues fully saturated with vitamin C. Although the levels were below normal they were above those found in people who developed scurvy. But, as Dr Nobile remarked: 'If an elderly person who is on a low intake of vitamin C develops an infection, the level can rapidly drop to a dangerous low and scurvy may develop.' The researchers believe that same old people are at risk because they are insufficiently educated in nutrition. They tend to buy the wrong foods, such as meat pies rather than fresh fruit. As well as this, those providing them with extra meals are also largely ignorant about nutrition. It is likely that this situation may also exist in other countries where dietary habits are similar to those in Australia but where fresh fruit and vegetables are even more expensive and often beyond the reach of the elderly, solitary poor.

Recently, Linus Pauling, Nobel Prizewinner in Biochemistry, has suggested that the recommended daily intake of vitamin C has resulted 'from a concentration by the authorities on the need to prevent scurvy' and that 'we should ask whether larger amounts might not be needed to provide an optimum state of health'. When a scientist of such distinction as Dr Pauling makes that sort of remark, one must review his evidence. In 1969 Drs Chaudhuri and Chatterjee had shown that most animals are able to synthesize vitamin C in their gut. Only man, other primates, the guinea-pig, the red-vented bulbul, and an Indian fruit-eating bat are unable to synthesize the vitamin and require ascorbic acid in their diet. Linus Pauling argues from this that somewhere in the several thousand million years of the evolution of living things, these animals lost their ability to synthesize ascorbic acid because they chose a diet which was rich in the vitamin. Man evolved from the great apes, and the great apes, during the millions of years of their evolution, were and are, vegetarian. They eat large quantities of leaves, fruits, grains, and nuts. Dr Pauling has calculated that great apes take in an average of 2,300 mg of ascorbic acid daily, and infers from his evolutionary argument that humans should take in a similar amount each day. If we did this, our state of health, 'including our ability to resist infection such as the common cold' would be greatly improved.

For many years a folk belief has existed that eating extra fruit will reduce the likelihood of catching colds, and Dr Pauling has made this folk belief scientifically respectable.

Linus Pauling's evolutionary hypothesis is difficult, if not impossible, to test because of the large gaps in the data. But it is possible to assess reasonably objectively whether an increased intake in vitamin C will prevent the common cold, which infects and causes suffering to millions of people each year. Dr Pauling claimed that if a person took 100 mg of ascorbic acid each day the incidence of colds would drop by about 45 per cent, and the total illness by 60 per cent. If vitamin C did prevent colds to this extent it would be a medical breakthrough of dramatic proportions, eclipsing almost any other of recent years. In most developed nations huge sums of money have been invested over the past 20 years into research to prevent the common cold, with monotonous and uniform lack of any positive results.

At the time when Dr Pauling wrote his paper, only four dependable double-blind studies had been reported. In these studies the effect of ascorbic acid in a daily dose of more than 100 mg was compared with a dose of a dummy sugar or citric acid tablet to see which group of people—those taking the vitamin or those taking the dummy—had the fewest colds, and if they did get a cold, whether it was less severe in one group or the other.

A major problem of this kind of investigation is that the definition of a cold is inexact, and is interpreted differently by different people. A second problem is that the duration of the trial differed in all four investigations and the dose of vitamin C was not identical. Dr Pauling was particularly attracted to the trial made in Switzerland by Dr Ritzel which involved 279 students at a ski-school and lasted a week. Dr Ritzel claimed that the students who took 1,000 mg of vitamin C each day had 45 per cent fewer colds than those taking the dummy tablets. The scientists conducting the other three investigations also reported that their results suggested that the people taking vitamin C had fewer colds, but the percentage differences between them and the controls were far less over the longer period of their investigations.

Dr Pauling enthusiastically supported his belief in a book *Vitamin C and the Common Cold*, published in 1970. The book had a wide popular appeal but also received a great deal of criticism from scientists and scientific writers.

Because colds are common and inconvenient and because of the amount of public interest aroused by Dr Pauling's book, groups of scientists in Britain, Canada, Ireland, and the U.S.A. have tried to answer two questions. These are, first: 'Will large daily doses of vitamin C reduce the frequency and duration of colds?'; and second, 'Does vitamin C make you feel better if you do catch a cold?'

To provide the answers the trials must extend for at least 90 days and large numbers of volunteers have to be involved. In addition the trials have to be 'double-blind'. This means that half of the volunteers have to take the dose of vitamin C recommended by Dr Pauling and half have to take an identical-looking capsule which contains no vitamin C. In the trials the capsules were taken each day and when the volunteer thought a cold was beginning, the number of capsules was increased considerably.

Eleven well-controlled trials involving 7,000 volunteers had been reported by 1979. These showed that the answer to the first question: 'Will large daily doses of vitamin C reduce the frequency and duration of colds' was a simple 'No!' In no trial did the volunteers taking vitamin C have fewer or shorter colds than the volunteers who took the capsules which contained only sugar.

The answer to the second question was a very doubtful 'Possibly!' In the second of the two Canadian trials conducted by Dr Anderson and his colleagues in Toronto, involving 2,400 volunteers for three months in the winter of 1973, large doses of vitamin C (4–8 g) taken as the cold started appeared to reduce the discomfort. In contrast the trial in the U.S.A. involving 311 volunteers made by Dr Karlowski and his colleagues, and that conducted by Dr Michael Carlson in Britain, did not show any difference in severity of or disability due to the cold even when large amounts of vitamin C were taken at the onset of the cold.

It seems from the evidence that vitamin C is useless in preventing a cold and probably of little value in reducing its severity. Moreover, large doses of vitamin C taken regularly may be harmful. Dr Michael Briggs of Melbourne, Australia, reports that large doses of vitamin C may precipitate demineralization of bones, cause the development of kidney stones, may reduce fertility in certain women, and may interfere with liver function, so masking the early signs of liver disease. These warnings about high dosages of vitamin C should be heeded.

Despite Dr Pauling's evolutionary approach, careful biochemical investigations have shown that a dose of 1,000 mg daily will produce complete saturation of the tissues, and any dose larger than this is simply excreted in the urine. In fact, the Canadian researchers who discovered this, Drs Spero and Anderson, wrote, 'In the present state of uncertainty we believe that a regular intake of more than 100–200 mg of vitamin C daily should be discouraged.' This view is supported by Dr Michael Briggs. In a letter to the *Medical Journal of Australia,* Dr Briggs wrote that the effectiveness of vitamin C in preventing colds was 'highly doubtful'. 'The only thing conclusively proven is that people who take large doses of the vitamin have a high excretory rate', said Dr Briggs. 'In fact they probably have the most expensive urine in the world.'

7

An insufficiency of energy, a paucity of protein

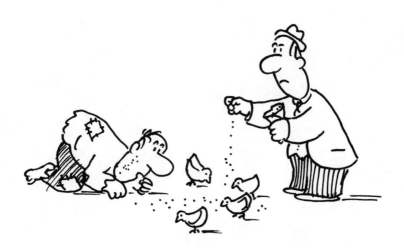

'Is there a protein gap? If one looks at figures for world and *per caput* availability of protein the answer is no . . . is there a protein problem? The answer is yes. The continuing high prevalence of protein–calorie malnutrition amongst children of the developing countries is prima facie evidence that suitable foods are not provided for such children, and, in many countries, that cultural practices deny young children sufficient access to protein foods.'   *Protein Advisory Group of the*
United Nations, Statement No. 20, 1973.

'. . . in the end the only real "gap" is the gap between the needs of an exploding world population and the provision to each individual of enough energy and balanced nutrients for his needs.'   *J. F. Brock, 1974.*

To those of us who live in the rich, developed, overfed third of the world, the problems of contemporary nutrition, with the exception of small minority groups, such as alcoholics and elderly, isolated people, are those of over-abundance. As I have tried to show in earlier chapters, many of the diseases common in the affluent nations are largely due to our lack of adaption to our new environment, and are aggravated by our over-indulgence in the wrong kinds of foods, or our dependence on drugs. The link between tobacco smoking and bronchitis, lung cancer, and heart disease is well established. Our over-indulgence in sugar is a factor in obesity, in dental decay, and in mature-onset diabetes, as I show in Chapter 4. The change in our diet to foods low in roughage (or perhaps a different type of roughage), is a factor in the increasing incidence of intestinal disorders. Excessive consumption of fats and sugars are probable factors in the 'epidemic' of heart disease occurring in rich nations.

The two-thirds of humanity who live in the hungry developing nations are largely spared these diseases, unless they belong to the upper 10 per cent of the population who tend to adopt a Western life-style. In contrast, the mass of humanity, and particularly the most vulnerable group—the children—are affected, often seriously, by undernutrition and by malnutrition. They eat too few calories to supply all their energy needs, so they are undernourished; and their diet contains too little protein, so they become malnourished.

The inter-relationship between insufficient energy (calorie) supply and protein lack has only been fully appreciated in recent years, and has led to the concept of protein–energy malnutrition. This disorder affects so many people that the United Nations has set up a special group of experts who meet regularly to consider the effects of protein–energy malnutrition and to suggest remedies.

In most parts of the world meat is a luxury only eaten on feast days and other special occasions; eggs are not eaten regularly, and cow's milk is not generally acceptable or obtainable. The diet of most people consists predominantly of cereals, and it is from the cereals (and the legumes which supplement the diet) that people have to obtain the energy and the protein they need. Protein is essential for the growth and repair of tissues. Consequently during periods of rapid growth rather more protein is required. This must be of a kind that contains all the essential amino-acids needed to create new tissues. A paucity of protein over this period can retard the growth and development of the person, can limit his 'capacity for achievement', and may have more serious consequences. A similar need for extra protein occurs at all ages during periods of tissue repair, such as after infectious illnesses.

Today's malnutrition is shackling tomorrow's generation of adults.

It is hardly surprising that studies by the United Nations indicate that perhaps as many as 500 million people are undernourished and that in many developing countries between 5 and 25 per cent of children suffer from protein–energy malnutrition.

Paradoxically, there is evidence that there is enough dietary protein available in the world to meet the daily protein needs of every man, woman, and child alive today, provided the protein foods could be distributed according to need. They are not. We, in the rich nations, eat far more protein than we need; so do the rich people in the poor nations. But in most of the developing nations, those groups who most need protein—pregnant women, children under the age of 5, and those suffering from infectious diseases—receive insufficient amounts, and because of food taboos may not be able to avail themselves of the protein that is available locally.

Protein–energy malnutrition affects between one-quarter and one-third of children under the age of 5 in many developing countries.

The conflicting arguments about protein availability have divided scientists into two separate camps. There are those who

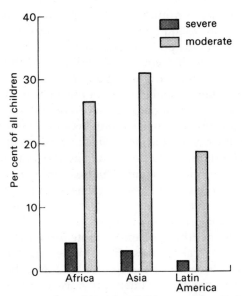

Protein-energy malnutrition in children under 5 in the under-developed continents

say that there is no protein shortage in the world, although there may be a shortage of food. They base their argument on United Nations statistics of protein production, and hold the opinion that in a satisfactory diet only 5–6 per cent of the energy needed has to be supplied by protein.

An example is given by Dr Bender, who is a proponent of this view. In 1967 statistics showed that Indonesia, with a *per capita* intake of protein averaging 38 g per day, had one of the lowest *per capita* intakes of protein. However, when the statistics were recalculated to find the percentage of total energy needs supplied by protein, the figure worked out at 7.7 per cent, a proportion which should give a person all the protein he needed provided the diet gave him all the calories he needed. From this, Dr Bender argued that in 1967, in Indonesia, the diet was short *neither* of energy nor of protein as such, but was short of food.

The scientists who oppose this relatively optimistic view (optimistic, that is, if you happen to be one of the well-fed third of mankind), do not deny the theoretical arguments, but say that in practice there is a serious protein shortage, which has occurred and which continues, because foods containing high quality protein are inequitably distributed between the rich affluent nations and the poor developing nations, between rich and poor families within countries, and even within households, where those who are most vulnerable to protein deficiency usually obtain a smaller share of the amount available.

In this situation, academic arguments become sterile, and it is largely irrelevant whether the diet contains sufficient protein if 5 per cent of the energy needed is supplied by protein, or whether the appropriate figure is 10 per cent. The fact is that a large number of people, mostly young children, are suffering, and often dying, because of protein–energy malnutrition. An insufficiency of energy and a paucity of protein is marring the lives of more than 500 million human beings in the world.

In practical terms, the problem of protein–energy malnutrition arises for several reasons. First, protein-rich foods are expensive, both because of the cost of land and the costs of production. The meat of animals provides a rich source of highly concentrated protein, but animals are expensive to rear and this aggravates the protein problem, because low wages and incomes, especially in the expanding towns of the developing world, severely limit the ability of most people to buy relatively costly protein-rich animal foods. Certain legumes are relatively rich in protein, compared with cereals, but legumes are becoming more expensive and there is an increasing trend away from legume to cereal production, which has been an unexpected result of the 'Green Revolution'.

It is true that with the introduction of new genetic strains of cereals (which is the essence of the 'Green Revolution'), the production per hectare of the grains has risen, and increasing hunger has been averted, if only temporarily. However, the grains have only been produced at a cost. They require complex agricultural techniques of precisely timed irrigation, fertilizer application, and pesticides. Irrigation depends on constantly available quantities of water and this in turn is dependent on energy to power the pumps. Fertilizer is produced from petrochemicals, and oil prices continue to rise. Moreover water and fertilizer nourish weeds as well as cereal plants, and the competition requires to be controlled in favour of the cereals by pesticides and constant weeding. Despite these criticisms, there is no doubt that the increased production of cereals has been beneficial and has made a significant impact in reducing potential hunger. It is also true that, provided sufficient amounts of cereals are eaten, supplemented by appropriate legumes, adults will be deficient in neither energy nor protein, as long as they avoid infectious diseases. This situation does not apply to young children. Cereal grains do not contain sufficient high quality protein, in the appropriate amino-acid mix, to meet a child's protein needs, especially if the child is prone to infections. The child *could* obtain sufficient protein if he could eat a large enough amount of cereal, but he doesn't because of its bulk. To this is added the problem of intestinal infection and parasites which limit the absorption of protein from the child's gut.

This problem is made worse if the total energy intake of the child is inadequate for its needs. When this occurs the child has to use most of the protein in its food to supply its energy needs, rather than reserving it for its proper function of repairing tissues.

The second reason for the continuing protein problem has already been mentioned. It is the inequitable distribution of protein-rich foods, when these are available, within households. All too often, because of a lack of knowledge of food values, or misguided methods of food preparation, or because of food prejudices, pregnant women and young children, the two most vulnerable groups, receive a disproportionately small share of protein-rich foods.

The third reason for the continuing protein problem in the Third World is that the solution of simply increasing the quantity of the traditional diet is not enough. Because of the cost of animal protein, and of taboos against weanlings and toddlers eating legumes or animal protein foods such as eggs, an increase in the traditional diet, although it is to be encouraged, may not in itself improve nutritional standards. Supplementary protein-rich foods must be added. And even if additional legumes are added to the diet, the child may prefer to eat the starchy cereals, so that the total intake needed to provide enough protein may be too bulky for the child to manage, unless the child is given five or six meals a day instead of the traditional two meals.

The extent of protein–energy malnutrition among pregnant and lactating women (the most vulnerable adult groups), among adults who have infectious diseases or have sustained injuries, and among young children, is difficult to gauge precisely. The Food and Agricultural Organization of the United Nations in 1969 found 'A widespread incidence of protein–energy malnutrition which affects one-quarter to one-third of children under the age of 5 in many of the developing countries for which data are available'. Underlying the careful use of these words is the human situation. This is that the majority of children in the world today, most of whom live in the developing nations, are not healthy. They suffer from frequent infections and most are malnourished. The food they eat provides a deficit in energy, which by comparison with their needs may be greater than the deficiency in protein, but both deficits are usually present.

The effects of this protein–energy deficiency may not be obvious at all, or they may appear as disease symptoms.

In younger children aged under 18 months, continuing protein–energy malnutrition (which begins after the child is weaned, and which is aggravated by repeated infections—usually diarrhoea), leads to a thin, wasted, miserable baby. It has nutritional marasmus (a word which means 'wasted'). It needs food to replace the energy and the protein it lacks.

In somewhat older children who have been breast-fed for a long period and are then weaned to eat the family diet, another type of protein malnutrition called kwashiorkor, may develop. The diet of the child who develops kwashiorkor may be adequate in energy but low in protein, or both the energy and protein may be deficient. In some situations, particularly in times of prolonged food shortage, this type of protein malnutrition may develop in children who are marasmic. In these children an episode of diarrhoea and respiratory infection leads to a sudden protein deficiency, either because protein is not being absorbed or because it is being burned up rapidly to counteract the infection. Kwashiorkor, the African name of the disease, means in the Ga language: 'the sickness that comes in the child that is weaned'. This accurately describes what happens. In mild kwashiorkor the child, already thin, develops a bloated swollen

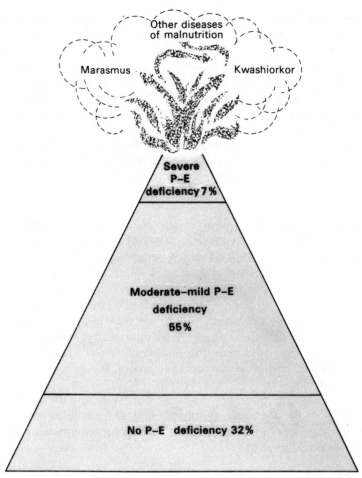

The 'volcano' of protein-energy malnutrition in the developing countries

belly and its hair has a reddish tinge. Suddenly, the child becomes very ill. It whines. It lies inert and apathetic, its legs swollen with fluid. Its hair falls out, its skin becomes dry, flaky, and patchily pale. It may develop severe diarrhoea. Unless it is treated quickly with protein supplements, preferably in the form of skimmed milk, it will die.

The relationship between the protein–energy malnutrition and infections, especially of the intestines, has frequently been observed, but has puzzled scientists for some time. Usually the child is relatively well so long as it is breast-fed, but once it is taken off the breast, problems arise.

Because it is no longer taking breast milk, the child has to eat the family diet as best it can. And because of cultural patterns and food taboos, it is unlikely to obtain sufficient food to meet its energy and protein requirements. Protein–energy malnutrition results.

It also becomes liable to suffer from frequent attacks of diarrhoea and other infections. These infections not only reduce the amount of food absorbed, but use up stored energy and protein because of the higher metabolic rate induced by fever. Malnutrition makes the child more liable to infection, which in turn aggravates the malnutrition. A vicious circle develops. A factor, recently determined by Professor Chandra in New Delhi, is that malnourished children have a reduced antibody response to infection, particularly of the antibody which is secreted into the nose and mouth and the rest of the gut. The secretory antibody, called immuno-globulin A, is known to produce a local immunity of cells lining the mouth, throat, and intestine, so that infections cannot get into the body. If that immunity is diminished, as it appears to be in malnutrition, infections are more likely to become established, and to be more severe. The vicious circle is perpetuated.

As I have discussed in Chapter 2, continued breast-feeding, at least to the age of six months, would do more to reduce the high number of infant deaths in developing nations than any other single measure.

In the developing countries of the world infant and childhood mortality is considerably higher than in the developed countries. The main reason for the higher mortality is the interaction between infectious diseases (especially viral diseases such as measles and poliomyelitis, and intestinal infections, mainly gastroenteritis) and protein–energy malnutrition. In many developing nations between one-quarter and one-third of all children born alive die in the first five years of life, compared with one or two in every hundred in the developed nations. After studying the data, experts from the FAO concluded that malnutrition was 'the biggest single contributor to child mortality in the developing nations' and that over 70 per cent of the 850 million children growing up in the developing countries might expect to 'encounter sickness or disabling disease either brought on or aggravated by protein–energy malnutrition'. Currently, although malnutrition is the *direct* cause of death in between only 3 and 10 per cent of child deaths under the age of 5, it is an *associated* cause in between 35 and 60 per cent of the deaths, since it affects the severity of measles, gastroenteritis, parasitic infection, and respiratory infections. It is likely that the figures are underestimated, since many deaths are not registered, or are registered inaccurately.

This appalling toll of life has its effect on family structure. Few families, expecting to lose one child out of every three born alive, are likely to respond favourably to the advice to use family planning to reduce the population growth rate. Yet, there is evidence that spacing children, using effective methods of birth control, will result in a better chance of survival for the existing children.

Mental retardation is only one of the threats of childhood malnutrition. Each year more than 15 million children under the age of 5 die because of the combined effects of malnutrition and infectious disease.

In laboratory experiments under controlled conditions, protein malnutrition of the mother in late pregnancy, or of the young in the early weeks of life, produced marked changes in the brains of the young of various experimental animals: rats, dogs, and pigs. In all these species, the brain size was much less in the protein-starved animals than in normal animals and, in addition, structural changes occurred in their brain cells. These findings suggest that malnutrition occurring during a critical stage of the growth of the brain could have lasting detrimental effects.

The brain is composed of two types of cells. The first are the nerve cells which multiply very early in foetal life. The second type of cells, called glial cells, proliferate later. The glial cells seem very important, because they help the nourishment of the

nerve cells and play an important role in communication between nerve cells at the nerve cell terminals. Dr Bernard Cragg,
who works in Monash University in Australia, found there were
40 per cent fewer nerve terminals in severely malnourished rats
than in infant rats whose mothers had not been starved. This
huge deficit would undoubtedly have had a terrible effect on
brain functioning.

These findings do not necessarily apply to all animals, particularly humans. Dr Donald Cheek, who also works in Melbourne, has studied the problem of maternal protein and calorie
malnutrition in the monkey *Macaca mulatta*. He was unable to
detect any damage to the brain cells of newborn monkeys
despite severe malnutrition during the pregnancy. These findings are important because monkeys are closer to humans in the
evolutionary ladder.

The critical time of brain growth varies between species. In
the pig it occurs during the period from five weeks before birth
to five weeks after birth. In the dog it is maximal during the 7–14
days after birth, while in the rat the critical time occurs during
the first ten days after birth.

It is, of course, impossible to apply the precise conditions of
controlled malnutrition that can be arranged for laboratory animals to humans, but it is worth finding out whether the brain
tissues and systems of human children react to protein–energy
malnutrition in a similar manner. What are the crucial periods of
time for this change to occur, if it does? And is the change
permanent, or can it be reversed?

The problems of answering these questions are great. In the
first place, protein-malnutrition in humans is never 'pure'; it is
allied to calorie lack, and both are often associated with
increased infection. All three may interfere with mother–child
contact and interaction. Secondly, children who suffer from
malnutrition are likely to come from homes in which other
deprivations—emotional, social, and stimulatory—are also
likely to be present. For these reasons a clear-cut answer to the
questions may be difficult to obtain.

In New York Dr Naeye investigated the effect of maternal
malnutrition during the last 10 weeks of pregnancy on the size
of the organs of nearly 500 babies dying before birth or during
the first days of life. He found that if the mothers were mal-

nourished, all of the child's organs were smaller, as was the size of the fat cells in its body, and the amount of adipose tissue was less. This suggested that undernourishment of the mother does affect the baby's tissues, perhaps including the brain.

In humans the peak rate of brain growth occurs at two specific times. The first period of rapid growth is in the last 3–4 weeks before birth and this period accounts for about one-sixth of human brain growth. The second period, when five-sixths of brain growth occurs, begins soon after birth, continues at this high level for six months, and lasts into the second year of life. In both of these phases, the main proliferation is of the glial cells.

There is limited evidence which suggests that malnutrition during either or both of the periods affects intellectual development, but good feeding in childhood may reverse some of the changes.

In Boston, U.S.A., a group of doctors, led by Dr Lloyd-Still, assessed the intellectual ability of 41 children who had severe malnutrition following intestinal disease in early infancy and compared each with a sibling (brother or sister) who was normal. The scientists found that the affected children had lower scores in intelligence tests, but after being given better nourishment over a period of years improved their scores so that they were similar to those of their siblings.

In Jamaica, a study of 74 boys who had been admitted to hospital with severe protein–energy malnutrition in the first two years of life was made by Dr Hertzig and her colleagues. They, too, found that the children who had been malnourished in early life were disadvantaged intellectually when compared with their normal siblings.

Both studies have defects which make the results obtained less clear and precise than might appear. For example, the Boston children with intestinal diseases were in hospital for long periods, and their mothers were alternately anxious or depressed. The poor intellectual functioning could therefore have been due to a general family disturbance. In the Jamaican investigation, although the 'control' child was the subject's brother closest in age to him, and a second control was a classmate or neighbour of similar age, Jamaican family structure is such that the brother could often have a different father, and the influence of stresses other than those due to malnutrition could not be excluded.

However, two recent reports from Africa suggest that children who suffer from chronic protein–energy malnutrition are permanently disadvantaged intellectually.

In South Africa a study has been made of the scholastic achievements of black African rural children who had suffered from severe protein–energy malnutrition during the first year of their life and 'control' children who were not chronically under-nourished. The investigation continued for over 21 years and the children were aged 15–18 at the time of the last report in 1976. The scientists, Drs Stoch and Smythe, have found that the severely malnourished children, despite improved environmental conditions and despite improved nutrition over the last 15 or so years, all have irreversible intellectual impairment, and their capacity to achieve has been reduced markedly.

Two other researchers, Drs Hoorweg and Stanfield, have come to the same conclusion. They studied the progress of 60 Ugandan children who had severe chronic protein–energy malnutrition (marasmus), and 60 children who did not have marasmus. By the age of 15 or more, the previously marasmic children were clumsier, less able to use words, less able to understand ideas, and had less over-all intellectual ability than the children who had not had marasmus. Their conclusion was that protein–energy malnutrition, which occurred in the first two years of life and continued for several months (so that the children were 'chronically undernourished') led to a permanent impairment of their intellectual ability.

While all nutritional scientists accept that intellectual status is the result of the interaction between malnutrition and other environmental factors, it appears that chronic protein–energy malnutrition exerts a sinister and permanent effect on the capacity for achievement of children who suffered from marasmus in early life.

Dr John Dobbing, a paediatrician in the Manchester Medical School, believes that more than 300 million children in the world may develop permanent intellectual defects because of malnutrition in early life. Most of these children live in the poor, hungry nations of the world. But even in our affluent, overfed countries, they are found in the slums of the big cities.

Nations that can develop a technology enabling them to send a space vehicle to orbit Mars, or to put a man on the moon; nations that can develop sophisticated destructive weaponry, can surely find the money and devote the time to prevent protein–energy malnutrition, and so enable the children of the Third World to reach their full potential. Is it too much to hope that mankind will turn its efforts away from expensive nationalistic posturing to the effort of preventing this waste of human achievement?

8

The fats of death?

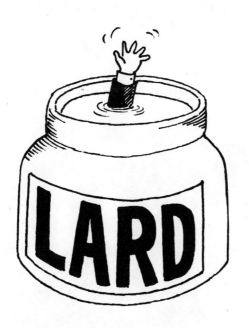

'Ischaemic heart disease (coronary heart disease) appears to have many contributory causes, and more than one is likely to be involved in determining the incidence of the disease in a population, or its occurrence in an individual. There is at present no evidence that any one cause has the essential importance for ischaemic heart disease which, for example, the tubercle bacillus has for tuberculosis.

Populations which have a high death rate from ischaemic heart disease have certain environmental features in common which appear to predispose them to the development of the disease. In any individual the liability to develop ischaemic heart disease is the result of an interaction between external risk factors and internal ones.'

Report of the Advisory Panel of the Committee on Medical Aspects of Food Policy on 'Diet in relation to Cardiovascular and Cerebrovascular Disease' (Department of Health and Social Security, United Kingdom, H.M.S.O., 1974).

Until the late 1960s in the U.S.A. and Australia, and a few years later in the developed nations of Europe, deaths from heart disease increased each year. Since that time there has been a 20 per cent reduction in the number of people (especially men) dying from acute heart attacks. Even so, in 1977 over 600,000 people in the U.S.A., 150,000 in Britain, 30,000 in Sweden, and 25,000 in Australia died as a result of coronary heart disease. To some extent the reduction in the deaths is due to better dietary habits and to a reduction in cigarette smoking; to some extent it is due to the better medical care available for the victim of an acute heart attack.

In spite of this gratifying improvement, coronary heart disease still kills one man in every 500 aged between 35 and 64. If a man in this age group has an acute heart attack he has a 30 per cent chance of dying within a few days, and most of those who die, do so within a few hours or minutes of the attack. Even if he is one of the 60 per cent who survive for a year, he has five times the chance of dying from a second heart attack in the next five years compared with a man who has not had an attack.

Although coronary heart disease was first described over 200 years ago, the disease was relatively uncommon until the last 50 years, especially in middle-aged people. The question that has to be asked is, Why has it become so common? To answer this question, you have to understand what leads to a heart attack, in other words, what causes coronary heart disease.

Scientists have found that coronary heart disease is a sudden, dramatic manifestation of a disease process that has been going on slowly in the arteries for a number of years. The process is called atherosclerosis of the arteries. The word atherosclerosis comes from two Greek words, *athere* and *sclerosis*. *Athere* means 'mush' or 'porridge'. The first pathologists who found mushy patches in the arteries of victims of heart attacks gave the patches a more distinguished name. *Sclerosis* means a firm narrowing. The entire word implies that certain parts of the affected artery are made narrower by a firm or mushy bulge.

Why the lining of these arteries becomes thickened in patches is unknown, but there is some recent evidence that either the blood pounding continuously along the artery, or some unknown blood substance, may start the process in susceptible people.

An artery is a flexible tube, and its wall has three layers. In childhood and early youth the innermost layer is thin, but as people grow older it becomes rather thicker. This inner layer is separated from the middle muscular layer by a band of elastic tissue, which is not complete, but has holes of various sizes in it. The outer layer of the artery is made up of fibrous tissue, rather like the fabric outer layer of an old fashioned hose-pipe.

One theory of how atherosclerosis starts is that the pounding blood irritates the lining of certain arteries, and substances (possibly released from blood platelets which stick to the damaged area) seep through the damaged wall. In some way these substances cause muscle cells from the middle layer to migrate through the holes in the elastic band and enter the inner layer. The migratory muscle cells are then stimulated to grow and reproduce, but they are also destroyed, and the balance between cell reproduction and destruction determines whether the inner layer thickens or becomes thinner. What determines this may be the level of fatty substances called lipids circulating in the blood, or the blood pressure, or perhaps the balance of sex hormones in the blood. The cause is not known.

If the lesion increases in size, lipids accumulate in the migratory muscle cells, and over the years the fat-containing muscle cells may increase in size and burst, releasing the fat into the surrounding tissue. This in turn causes a body reaction and a scar-tissue scaffold is built up through the damaged area and between the fat-containing cells.

At first fatty dots or thin fatty streaks (as the World Health Organization calls them) appear beneath the inner lining of the arteries. These fatty streaks can appear remarkably early in life. For example, Dr Enos and his colleagues found them in 12 per cent of American soldiers killed in the Korean War on whom they performed autopsies, and similar findings were made in Chile by Dr Viel and his colleagues when autopsies were made on young men who had died violently. An even more disturbing finding was made in New Orleans, where fatty streaks were found in the aortas of a large number of children who were three years old or less when they died, and they were found in the coronary arteries of nearly all those who had died at the age of 20.

It seems that fatty dots and streaks occur early in life and represent the beginning of a process which may lead to atherosclerosis. It is also probable that the fatty streaks can disappear, given certain changes in a person's life-style. The problem is that there is no way of knowing which alternative will occur.

If they are going to progress, the fatty streaks increase in size over the years, and by the time a person is in his late twenties or early thirties, they will have become patches; usually circular in shape, which bulge to a greater or lesser degree into the cavity of the artery. This condition is atherosclerosis.

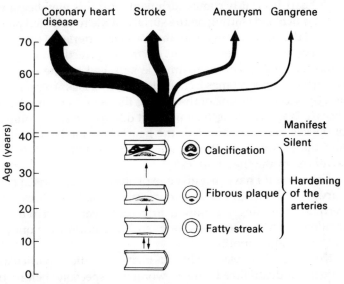

Hardening of the arteries (atherosclerosis)

If a person who has atherosclerotic arterial disease dies, an autopsy will show the creamy, lipid-containing patches along the affected arteries. The main lipids deposited are cholesterol and triglycerides. At first the lipids are deposited in the muscle cells which have migrated into the damaged innermost layer of the artery but, in the later stages, crystals of cholesterol are deposited between the cells. Cholesterol is thought by many scientists to be the most important lipid in the process, because it prevents other lipids from becoming emulsified and then disappearing. Some scientists believe that the cholesterol crystals are only deposited between the cells when the level of lipids in the blood is high; while the lipid in the cells is not related to blood lipid level.

Provided the thickened patch has a smooth covering on its inner side, which is the lining of the artery, it causes little trouble until advanced old age, when the thickening of the arteries to the brain may prevent an adequate flow of blood with a resultant loss of mental ability. But if the lining becomes invaded by the cholesterol crystals, its surface becomes roughened. As the blood pounds past the roughened area with each heart-beat, it becomes turbulent, and this may begin the process of blood clotting on the surface of the roughened patch. Should the clot occur in one of the coronary arteries of the heart, the person has a 'heart attack' or, more correctly, a coronary artery occlusion. The heart muscle supplied by the occluded coronary artery becomes ischaemic, that is, it lacks oxygen, and as a consequence some of the muscle fibres die. This is why the disease is also called ischaemic heart disease. If a large number of muscle fibres are affected, the heart ceases to beat properly and the person dies. If only a few are affected the victim recovers from the 'heart attack'.

The account I have just given explains *what* happens in coronary heart disease, but it does not explain *why* heart disease has become increasingly common in recent years, and why the incidence of atherosclerosis varies so dramatically from one part of the world to another.

Nor does it explain why in many societies (particularly affluent industrialized ones), women, especially before the menopause, are less likely to have coronary heart disease than men of a similar age. It has been suggested that the female sex hormones in some way protect women, since after the menopause when the sex hormone level drops, women and men have an almost equal chance of developing heart disease. Unfortunately for this theory, there is evidence that women of non-white races living in poor nations, both before and after the menopause, develop heart disease as frequently as men.

From the huge quantity of reports, papers, books, speculations, conferences, 'on-going' studies, longitudinal multiphasic analyses, and guesses, the only real conclusion is that several 'risk factors' are implicated in this disease of affluent man. Scientists define 'risk factors' as those habits, or inherited traits, which at least double the chance of a person developing coronary heart disease before the age of 65. The risk factors are raised blood cholesterol (due to present day dietary preferences), cigarette smoking, high blood pressure, lack of exercise, obesity, and perhaps stress. The problem is to determine from the contradictory evidence which of the risk factors is the most important, or whether all are of equal importance.

It is generally accepted that atherosclerosis is very rare in the developing world, unless Western dietary habits and life-styles are adopted. One way of investigating this is to compare the death rate due to atherosclerosis in men aged 40–59, in various parts of the world.

For such a study to be valid, the diagnosis of the cause of death needs to be accurate. In general this means that an autopsy has been made. Autopsies on elderly people in developing countries are not usual, but in 1972 Dr Drury, who was working at that time in Uganda, reported on autopsies of 373 Ugandans aged 60 or over. Among these men he found that only 6, or 1.6 per cent, had atherosclerosis. This incidence is nearly 20 times less than among white men of a similar age.

In most developing countries autopsies are unobtainable, as are reports from death certificates. However, some clinical studies have been made by careful observers. These show that among the Masai and the Samburu in East Africa and among the Bantu in South Africa atherosclerosis is rare, as it is among other Africans who live a tribal life. Once the Africans move to the towns coronary heart disease becomes more common, until it is almost as common as among white men living in the towns. There is a clue here to the cause, or causes of atherosclerosis. The problem is, what is the clue? Is atherosclerosis due to a dietary change, or to a change in the way of life, or to something else?

The evidence from a large number of studies suggests that atherosclerosis is brought about in susceptible individuals by life-long bad eating habits, but that a certain life-style plays a considerable, if secondary, part in the end result of atherosclerosis—a heart attack.

Field surveys in many countries throughout the world show that in places where a large amount of fat, and a large quantity of refined carbohydrate (especially sugar) is eaten, coronary heart disease is particularly common. It is possible to draw a graph in which the quantity of fat in the diet is correlated with the proportion of deaths from coronary heart disease.

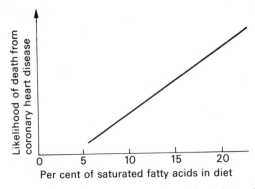

How fat in the diet increases the risk of dying from
coronary heart diseases

It is also possible to relate the quantity of refined sugar in the diet to the fat in the diet. You can see that the more fat in the diet, the greater the chance of coronary heart disease occurring; and people who eat a lot of fat also eat a lot of sugar. This finding is not entirely unexpected, as the more affluent the community the more money the people spend on meat and dairy products and on sugar. Quite often, too, in Western diets, fats, and sugars are mixed in a cooked food. This occurs in cakes, biscuits, puddings, sauces and chocolate.

In this regard, the documented changes in eating habits in Britain and the U.S.A. may be relevant. In the U.S.A., since about 1890, there has been a steady decline in the total amount of carbohydrate eaten, but a steady increase in the proportion due to consumption of sugar. In Britain there was a sharp drop in carbohydrate consumption until about 1910, after which the level became stable, but the stability was due to an increase in the consumption of refined sugar. If the ratio between complex carbohydrates (found in wholemeal flour and vegetables) and simple carbohydrates (usually refined sugar, including the sugar content of manufactured foods, honey, and glucose) is calculated, the ratio has decreased sharply in both countries. In other words, people today eat less unrefined carbohydrate in their diets, but more refined sugar than they did 75 years ago. Over the same period people have increased the quantity of protein they eat, but the amount of fat has only increased slightly, at least in the U.S.A., and most of the increase has been in polyunsaturated fats.

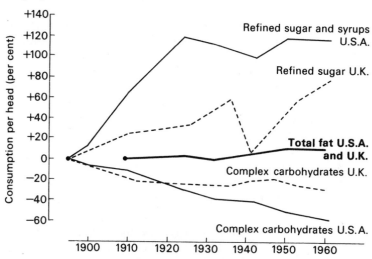

Changes in the consumption of carbohydrates and fats in the U.S.A. and the U.K. since 1895

The case against fats

Every housewife knows what she means when she buys fat: she means butter, margarine, or lard, or she means the fat on (or in) the meat she buys. She doesn't mean the fat she and her family eat, because fat is 'hidden' in most foods, ranging from nearly 40 per cent of the weight of the food in many cheeses, in potato chips, and in chocolate, to a mere trace in most vegetables and fruits. Hidden fat is also contained in cakes, in biscuits, in puddings, and in sauces.

Fats provide a concentrated source of energy, but are indigestible in quantity (unless you are an Eskimo!). Fats improve the taste of food and, in the diet which we choose to eat in the developed nations, provide over 40 per cent of our daily energy (calorie) intake.

When a biochemist talks about fats, he uses the term lipids. Lipids in the diet are formed from fatty acids linked with other substances in various ways, usually as triglycerides, phospholipids, or cholesterol.

The fatty acids that make up the lipids may be saturated or unsaturated, and the proportion between the two varieties in the diet is thought to play a role in the development of coronary heart disease. Saturated fatty acids are mainly found in animal fats or dairy products, but one vegetable fat is highly saturated. This is coconut oil which is used in tropical areas for cooking and in Western nations as a base for ice-cream manufacture. Unsaturated fats, particularly polyunsaturated fats, are usually vegetable in origin and are obtained mainly from sunflower oil, safflower oil, corn oil, and olive oil (though olive oil is in fact monounsaturated). Fish is another source of polyunsaturated fats.

The form in which fats chiefly occur, both in the food you eat and in the fat stored in your body, is in triglycerides, which are made up from three fatty acids and glycerol. Cholesterol is found in a number of foods, particularly egg yolk, but only forms a small part of the fat you get in your diet, because it is not readily absorbed. Most of the cholesterol in your blood is manufactured in your body, but recent evidence shows that a proportion is absorbed from cholesterol in the diet, and the quantity absorbed seems to be increased by the amount of saturated fatty acids in your diet. The one helps the other. The more saturated fatty acids in the diet, the more of the cholesterol in the diet is absorbed. It has also been found that the more fats that are absorbed from the diet, the more cholesterol is mobilized from the liver (where it is manufactured), and the more cholesterol enters the blood-stream. Conversely, there is evidence that the higher the proportion of polyunsaturated (vegetable) fats in the diet, the less cholesterol is absorbed from the gut, the less is mobilized from the liver, and the more is excreted in the urine and faeces. You will recall that cholesterol is the substance found in the patches on the walls of the arteries of those persons who have atherosclerosis, so the importance of these observations is obvious.

The question which has to be answered is this: Does a persistent high blood cholesterol (more accurately a serum cholesterol) produce atherosclerosis, or is it a chance finding? One way to find out would be to take two groups, and feed one a diet rich in fats and cholesterol, and to feed the other group a diet which contained no fats or cholesterol. Obviously it would be considered unethical to conduct such an experiment on humans, so laboratory animals are chosen.

Dr Scott and his colleagues in the U.S.A. used pigs as the experimental animal, since in many respects their eating habits are similar to those of man! They will eat virtually anything, and atherosclerotic lesions appear spontaneously in pigs fed on swill. Dr Scott fed the pigs a variety of fatty diets for periods varying from 30 to 330 days, and compared them with pigs fed on an ordinary stock diet. The pigs eating a diet rich in saturated fats and cholesterol began to develop fatty streaks after 30 days, and by 330 days they had severe atherosclerosis in their aortas. When the scientists took pieces of aortas and looked at them under a microscope, they found lesions identical with the atherosclerotic lesions found in man. When they measured the level of cholesterol in the pigs' blood, they found that those pigs who had the most advanced atherosclerosis also had the highest levels of serum cholesterol.

Perhaps a more conclusive experiment was carried out on animals closer to man in the evolutionary scale—monkeys. Dr Connor and his team of scientists fed rhesus monkeys on a diet rich in cholesterol and fats for 17 months and found that a large number of monkeys developed atherosclerosis. He then gave the monkeys a low-fat, low-cholesterol diet which was rich in polyunsaturated fats, and found that the fatty patches in the arteries disappeared.

The conclusion reached from various similar experiments was that in chickens, rabbits, dogs, and monkeys, a high serum-cholesterol level was produced by a diet rich in saturated fatty acids and cholesterol, and that some time later most of the animals developed atherosclerosis. The problem with all these investigations was that the diets chosen were grossly abnormal for the animals, and would not normally be eaten by man. And, of course, none of the experiments proved that these diets would cause atherosclerosis in man.

Dietary experiments on humans are extremely difficult to arrange. Not only do humans fail to keep to the diet, but the additional factors which may contribute to heart disease—cigarette smoking, sedentary occupations, high blood pressure, and stress—vary so much in different people that controls are difficult to obtain. Moreover the trials have to continue over a long period of time.

However, some studies are in progress which seek to find answers to the following questions: Does a diet containing a large quantity of animal fats lead to a high blood level of cholesterol (called hypercholesterolaemia), and does this, over a period of time, lead to atherosclerosis in certain blood vessels?

To answer this question, two types of trial have been set up. In the first, the scientists wanted to see if special diets, which were low in saturated animal fats, were better able to prevent coronary heart disease than a 'normal' diet. In the second trial, the scientists wanted to find out if a special diet altered the course of the disease in survivors of heart attacks. Two well-organized, well-designed, and well-controlled trials have attempted to answer the second question. One was under the guidance of Professor Leren in Oslo, and the other was organized by Professor Morris in London. Both investigations were made on about 400 men who had had a heart attack—a coronary thrombosis. Half of each group ate a special diet in which the fat was mostly polyunsaturated soybean oil; the other half ate an ordinary diet. In the Oslo investigation fewer of the experimental group—16 per cent—had a second heart attack than the men in the ordinary diet group, 27 per cent of whom had a further attack; and the attack among the group on an ordinary diet was three times more likely to be fatal. In the English study, 22 per cent of the men on the special diet had a relapse compared with 25 per cent of those on an ordinary diet. The Oslo investigation suggested that diet did help to reduce the risk of further heart attacks; the English investigation suggested that diet made little difference.

Trials set up to determine whether diet can prevent heart attacks are very difficult to conduct because so few people are prepared to follow the dietary recommendations strictly over a long period. However, one trial reported in 1972 from Finland provides suggestive evidence about the influence of saturated fat on heart disease, although some reservations have been expressed about the design of the trial. In it, patients in two mental hospitals were given diets that were only slightly different. In one hospital ordinary milk was replaced by an emulsion of soybean oil in skimmed milk (called 'filled milk'), and butter was replaced by polyunsaturated margarine. As well as this, the amount of sugar in the experimental diet was reduced from about 100 g daily to 60 g daily. Apart from these changes, the diets were similar. After six years the hospital which had provided the special low-saturated diet changed to the ordinary diet and the hospital which had provided the ordinary diet changed to the special diet. Over the 12 years of study various measurements were made on blood samples taken from the patients and an autopsy was made on each person who died. Dr Miettinen and the other scientists concluded that the blood cholesterol of men eating the special diet was between 10 and 20 per cent lower than when they ate the ordinary diet and the chances of them dying from coronary heart disease were halved. In women the findings were less consistent, but the same trend was discerned.

The reservations about this experiment are that the two groups were constantly changing as patients were discharged and new patients were admitted, and that the observers may have been biased about the results they expected.

The best reported and most exhaustive study of the effect of dietary fats, particularly cholesterol, on the development of coronary heart disease has been made in the city of Framingham, Massachusetts. A group of 2,282 men and 2,845 women aged 30–62 when first examined, and found to be free from heart disease, have been followed up for over 20 years. Eighty per cent of the original group are still being medically examined every two years, and 8 per cent have died. Information about their health has been obtained from another 10 per cent, and fewer than 2 per cent have not been traced. This is a remarkable achievement and shows the motivation and interest of the people of Framingham, and the respect with which they regard the medical scientists who conduct the study.

At each of the examinations blood specimens are examined for lipids, especially cholesterol, and any suspected episode of coronary heart disease is fully investigated, before a firm diagnosis is made.

In 1971 Dr Kannel and his colleagues reported on the first 14 years of study. During these years 323 men and 169 women had developed heart disease. The disease became more common as the people grew older, as might be expected. The younger the victim was, the more likely it was to be a man, but the gap closed with age when both sexes became equally, or nearly equally, prone to heart attacks.

A significant observation, which supports the case against fats, was that the risk of a heart attack was proportional to the concentration of each of the lipids measured, and cholesterol was the most important lipid. The higher the level of serum cholesterol, at each examination, the higher the risk that the individual would develop coronary heart disease. If the serum cholesterol was more than 265 mg per 100 ml of serum, the individual had two to five times the chance of developing coronary heart disease than if it was below 220 mg per 100 ml, and the younger the individual the greater the risk. This meant that if the man or woman whose blood cholesterol was 265 mg per 100 ml or higher was under the age of 45, he or she had 5 times the chance of a heart attack than a person whose serum cholesterol was under 220 mg per 100 ml. By the time the man reached 50, the risk was only twice as high, and a woman of 50 who had a high blood cholesterol had only a slightly increased risk of developing a heart attack.

The Framingham scientists were unable to decide whether the serum cholesterol level was determined by genetic factors, such as having a father who had a high serum cholesterol, or by over-eating, but they felt that the latter was the more important.

In practical terms, most recent research, particularly the Framingham study, does point to the fact that if a person under the age of 50 has a serum cholesterol of less than 200 mg per 100 ml he is very unlikely to have a heart attack, but if his serum cholesterol is more than 260 mg per 100 ml he is increasingly at risk of coronary heart disease. In other words, hypercholes-terolaemia (that is, too high a level of cholesterol in the blood serum) is associated, in some way, with atherosclerosis. This raises the question: If the serum cholesterol is lowered by diet or drugs, will the chances of a heart attack be reduced?

American scientists have tried to answer this question, but with only limited success. They have followed a number of volunteers who have reduced their daily intake of cholesterol from the usual 600 mg a day in the average American diet to 300 mg a day, and their consumption of saturated animal fats from 40 per cent to 35 per cent of all fats eaten, by eating a diet in which polyunsaturated margarine is substituted for butter, eggs are eaten sparingly, bacon eaten rarely, milk and cheese are limited, and ice-cream is only eaten on special occasions. Their conclusion was that on this type of diet, the blood cholesterol levels would be reduced by 10 per cent, and the risk of having a heart attack would be reduced by 24 per cent.

The findings of the American studies have been criticized by biological scientists and by statisticians. The biologists have pointed out that a single estimation of serum cholesterol (which was used) should be interpreted with great caution, as many factors can influence the level. The statisticians noted that none of the American studies necessarily represented the American population: neither upper nor lower socio-economic groups were properly represented. They also observed that nearly one-third of the people dropped out of the studies, and that when the information was re-analysed, tobacco smoking appeared to be a more serious risk factor than a high blood cholesterol level, which was assumed to be due to American eating preferences.

A reason for the inconclusive findings about the benefit of manipulation of the diet to reduce cholesterol intake may be that scientists have been measuring the wrong substance.

Scientists have recently found that cholesterol is transported in the body by two 'carrier' lipoproteins. The first, low-density lipoprotein (LDL), attaches to cholesterol and transports it to body cells, where it is involved in helping repair cell walls. The second, high-density lipoprotein (HDL), is able to remove excess cholesterol from cells and transport it to the liver, where it is stored. The scientists have also found that only cholesterol attached to LDL can seep through the damaged lining of arteries to be taken up by the muscle cells which have migrated there. These findings have been applied to people with coronary heart disease. Doctors have discovered that if the level of HDL-cholesterol in your blood is low and that of LDL-cholesterol is high you have an increased risk of coronary heart disease. When doctors only measured total serum cholesterol this important distinction was obscured.

The case against dietary fats is still not fully proved, but the evidence is sufficiently strong for people, especially men, to beware of eating too much cholesterol (eggs, kidneys) and too many saturated animal fats (marbled red meat and butter).

The case against sugar

Although most scientists studying coronary heart disease agree that the quantity and type of fatty foods eaten influences the level of serum cholesterol, which in turn is a factor in heart disease, some believe that the amount of sugar in the diet is also important. These scientists point out, for example, that Eskimos eat a diet which consists mainly of fatty meat, eating up to 3 kg of meat a day, when they can get it. They eat hardly any carbohydrate or sugar. In spite of this diet, which is rich in saturated fats, an investigation in the Aleutian Islands by Dr Alexander showed that coronary heart disease was very rare in Eskimos. Heart disease is also rare among the rural Bantu living in Natal, but becomes more common amongst Africans living in towns. When Dr Campbell investigated the diet of the two groups, he found that the only real difference was that the rural Bantu ate very little sugar (less than 6 g a day) compared with the urban Bantu who were eating increasing amounts, and were rapidly catching up with the white African's daily intake of 60 g.

Further north in East Africa, as I mentioned earlier in this chapter, the Masai and the Semburu tribes, and other cattle-economy tribes, drink at least 5 litres of milk a day, and eat meat. That is their whole diet. They eat no sugar, and few carbohydrates. Despite this high fat diet, their blood cholesterol is low, and coronary heart disease is unknown.

An interesting piece of evidence was obtained by Dr Cohen

and his colleagues in Israel. They studied the diet of the black Jews from the Yemen before they left their homeland, and compared it with the diet they adopted after their repatriation to Israel. In the Yemen, the black Jews mainly ate animal meat, which had a high content of mutton and beef fat, and very little sugar. In Israel, there was a startling ten-fold increase in their sugar consumption, but little increase in their fat consumption, their protein consumption, or the total number of calories they ate each day. About ten years after repatriation, the black Jews began to have heart attacks, which they said rarely occurred when they lived in the Yemen, and which were unknown among new Yemeni settlers in Israel. Dr Cohen concluded that the high intake of sugar (which rose from about 7 g to 63 g a day) had something to do with it.

It is also known that diabetic individuals have a high risk of developing coronary heart disease. The reason may have been found by a pathologist, Dr Siperstein. He has made very careful examinations of small blood vessels in the muscles of diabetics, of unaffected children of diabetic parents, and of non-diabetics using an electron microscope. These studies show that the lining of the vessels (actually it is the basement membrane) is thickened in more than 98 per cent of diabetics, in 53 per cent of the relatives of diabetics, but in only 8 per cent of non-diabetics. Dr Siperstein claims that the blood vessel thickening is even more important in diabetes than is the impaired insulin response to a glucose drink or to an injection of glucose. And, as I mentioned earlier in this chapter, changes in the walls of blood vessels are thought to be important in atherosclerosis.

The person who develops diabetes in middle life, often after years of over-eating refined carbohydrates and sugar, tends to be overweight and has an increased risk of premature atherosclerotic disease, either in his aorta, his coronary arteries, in the arteries supplying his brain, or in the arteries of his legs. This association has been found in many studies, notably in one involving 73,000 men and women aged 25–64 employed by the Dupont company. In this and other studies in the U.S.A., the higher risk of heart disease extended to people who did not have clinical diabetes, but whose blood sugar when tested after a meal was higher than usual.

These findings add support to the suggestion that in some

way too much sugar in the diet, over the years, adds to the effect of too much saturated fat, and is a risk factor in coronary heart disease.

Although studies of populations suggest that sugar may be a factor in heart disease, the experimental evidence is less conclusive. In Sweden, Dr Malmros and his colleagues fed a group of rabbits on a diet, nearly half of which was made up of sugars and starch, but which contained no cholesterol or fat. After some time, Dr Malmros measured the blood cholesterol levels of the rabbits. Those whose diets consisted mainly of starch showed no change in the cholesterol levels of their blood, but if the rabbits were given sucrose or glucose a small rise did occur. However, when the experiment ended after one year, and the animals were killed and examined, only those animals which had been fed sucrose showed any atherosclerotic areas in their aortas, and even these were not very marked.

In humans, the problems of conducting a reliable investigation are enormous. Professor Yudkin, who believes that sugar is a major risk factor, found that if large amounts of sucrose were eaten by men (427 g a day compared with the average English consumption of 142 g a day) the blood cholesterol levels, the triglyceride levels and the stickiness of the platelets in the blood all increased significantly. In this he is, in part, supported by Dr Epstein who has been studying the effect of diet on blood cholesterol levels, and on the incidence of heart disease, for over ten years in a community living at Tecumseh in Michigan. Dr Epstein found that in the vulnerable 40–59 age group, high blood cholesterol levels and heart attacks were associated among men; but he also found men and women who had high blood sugar levels were more likely to die from coronary disease. Amongst the people of Tecumseh the risk of coronary heart disease occurring in a man aged 25–64 was two and a half times greater than average if he had diabetes. In Sweden, Dr Wahlberg reported in 1966 that when survivors of heart attacks were examined during their recovery period, a very large number showed abnormally high blood sugar levels after eating a meal containing 100 g of sugar. And at about the same time an almost identical finding was reported from Natal in South Africa among the survivors of coronary heart disease. These men were of Indian origin.

These observations suggest that a high sugar intake may increase the person's blood level of triglyceride and that this may increase the risk of heart disease. A high sugar intake may also operate in another way. Scientists have found that diets rich in sugar (and refined carbohydrates) reduce the level of the 'protective' HDL-cholesterol.

At present, in spite of the research, and the considerable contributions made by Professor Yudkin and his colleagues, most investigators have failed to find an association between high intake of refined carbohydrates in the diet and subsequent coronary heart disease. But too much sugar and other refined carbohydrates does lead to obesity and, in susceptible people, to diabetes. Both of these conditions may predispose to coronary heart disease.

The case against cigarette smoking

In the United States, Britain, and Australia there is increasing evidence that cigarette smoking is an important factor in causing coronary heart disease.

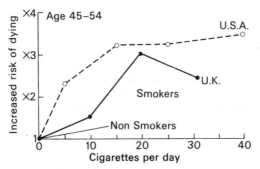

How cigarette smoking increases the risk for middle-aged men of dying from coronary heart diseases

Between 1959 and 1967 Drs Hammond and Garfinkle investigated over one million men and women aged 40–79. They found that men aged 40–49 who smoked more than 20 cigarettes a day had four times the chance of having a heart attack compared with non-smokers. Similar studies in Britain confirmed the association between cigarette smoking and heart attacks. For example, Sir Richard Doll and Dr Peto reported in 1977 on a 20-year study of the smoking habits of doctors. Men under the age of 45 who smoked 25 or more cigarettes a day had 15 times the chance of having a heart attack compared with non-smokers. As the doctors grew older the difference in heart attacks between smokers and non-smokers diminished, but a difference remained.

That is the bad news. The good news is that if you give up cigarette smoking, your increased risk of heart disease diminishes, and after 3–5 years it is no greater than that of non-smokers.

Scandinavian scientists also confirm that cigarette smoking is a major risk in coronary heart disease. Dr Werko re-examined three American studies and came to this conclusion. Dr Holme and his colleagues in Oslo noted that coronary heart disease was more common in people in lower socio-economic groups who ate substantially similar diets but smoked more cigarettes than people in the higher socio-economic groups.

Why cigarette smoking should be involved in the cause of coronary heart disease has puzzled scientists for some time. The connection has seemed remote. Or it was until recently when a joint investigation by medical investigators in Oxford and in Copenhagen partly answered this question. Dr Knud Kjeldsen had noticed that raised blood levels of carbon monoxide in animals led to atherosclerosis, and he wondered if smoking, which is known to raise blood carbon monoxide, might have a similar effect in humans. In a study of over 1,000 people Dr Kjeldsen found that it did. A heavy smoker aged 30–60 years old, with a blood carbon monoxide level (due to inhaling tobacco smoke) of 5 per cent or more, had over 20 times the chance of developing coronary heart disease compared with a light smoker, or a non-smoker, who had a blood carbon monoxide level of 3 per cent or less.

The case against sloth

Lack of exercise has been considered a cause of coronary heart disease in recent years, but this assumption must be questioned. If lack of exercise is a cause of heart attacks, it is presumably also a cause of atherosclerosis of the coronary arteries, for these precede heart attacks. With increasing evidence that the first fatty streaks appear in childhood or adolescence, at a time when physical activity is usual, it is difficult to understand how lack of exercise can be implicated. It is also unlikely that lack, or excess, of exercise is in any way implicated in any of the theories of the origin of atherosclerosis. If the patches in the arteries form because of high levels of serum cholesterol which somehow permit the lipids to seep through the arterial wall, how could exercise be implicated, for exercise has not been shown to affect the level of the lipids or the permeability of the arterial wall? If they form because of the stickiness of blood platelets, once again there is no evidence that exercise has any material effect.

In fact, one could speculate that once the plaque had formed, exercise might be harmful, at least in theory; the more rapidly circulating blood would pound on the smooth surface of the plaque and might more easily cause it to rupture, thus initiating a blood clot.

However, Dr Ward of Stanford University in California found that the blood levels of cholesterol and other lipids are lower among men who exercise regularly. Regular exercise also has a direct effect on a person's heart. The heart of a man who exercises regularly beats at a slower rate and responds to sudden exertion by increasing its rate to a smaller degree. It is a more efficient heart, and one study has shown that coronary arteries are larger in the hearts of men who exercise regularly. These changes may help in preventing 'heart attacks'.

It is sensible for people, in our largely sedentary civilization, to exercise more. It can be quite painless. Walk to the shops, walk up the stairs of buildings, and avoid the lifts. The kind of exercise you do must be one you enjoy. If you enjoy jogging, then jog. If you hate jogging, do some other exercise. Actively garden, or play energetic golf (that means you walk briskly around the course), swim, or ride a bicycle. It is unwise to take violent, unaccustomed exercise—such as squash once a week—and far better to take regular exercise.

At a meeting of heart specialists held in Los Angeles, California, in 1972, the eminent and erudite Emeritus Professor of Cardiology, Dr George C. Griffeth, remarked, 'I have never advised individuals to jog if they have not been in the habit of regular exercise. I jogged or ran four miles every day for about

30 years and enjoyed it because it gave me time to be with my dogs and it provided a sense of well-being. I do not know how much benefit was derived since it did not prevent a coronary attack', he added ruefully.

This attitude is supported in part by an investigation in Ireland in 1975. The scientists were anxious to find out if physical activity at work and during leisure bore any relationship to the risk of coronary heart disease. The odd result of the investigation of the sloth or the activity of more than 15,000 Irishmen was that exertion at work did not protect against heart attacks but leisure activity did. The conclusion Dr Hickey and his colleagues reached was that those men who took more exercise in their leisure time were more likely 'to smoke less and eat more prudently for personality, psychological, or cultural reasons'. In other words physical exercise itself did not reduce the risk of heart disease.

This is just about what Dr Griffeth had said, but that doesn't mean that exercise is not beneficial to a person. A person who enjoys exercise is less likely to gorge himself, to smoke heavily, and to be under stress. And stress may be a risk factor in heart disease.

The case against obesity

Two further factors are believed to be involved in accelerating the onset of heart attacks. These are obesity and high blood pressure. Obesity is a result of eating more calories than are required for the daily activity of the person. These excess calories are derived mainly from carbohydrates, and to a lesser extent, from fat. It should be said that overweight *alone* is not a factor in premature heart attacks—as many thin men as fat men suffer from coronary heart disease, according to Dr Keys who has been studying heart disease for over 20 years.

Dr Key's findings do not exclude the possibility that overeating contributes to the epidemic of coronary heart disease found in affluent Western societies. The evidence indicates that it does, but the association is neither simple nor direct.

In Chapter 1, I showed that in our overfed societies most men and women can expect to gain between 9 and 12 kg in weight in the 20 years after reaching maturity. In other words they can expect to be 9–12 kg heavier at the age of 45 than they were when they were aged 20–25. As so many people gain this amount of weight, many physicians accept it as normal and conclude that the amount of weight gained is of little significance in the development of coronary heart disease. This opinion is probably incorrect, and the weight gain in maturity, which is mainly due to over-indulgence in sugar, alcohol, and refined cereals, probably has an indirect effect which increases the likelihood of a heart attack.

It is accepted by most heart specialists that high blood levels of triglycerides and of cholesterol do increase the risk of coronary heart disease and such levels are found in certain susceptible people who have over-eaten in the 20 years or so after they have reached maturity. In fact, a recent finding from the Tecumseh study (see p. 164) suggests that a person's blood level of cholesterol and triglycerides depends more on his obesity than on the quantity of saturated fats or refined carbohydrates he has eaten over the years.

In the belief that the blood levels of triglycerides and of cholesterol could be reduced by dieting alone, Professor Blacket and his colleagues in Sydney, Australia, sought the help of the Australian Red Cross Blood Bank. Blood donors in Australia are checked before they give blood. One check measures the levels of their blood lipids (or fats), which include cholesterol and the triglycerides. In 1970–71, one hundred healthy blood donors were found to have high blood levels of triglycerides. Twenty of the men agreed to co-operate with Professor Blacket. After discussions, the men agreed to stop over-eating and to go on a diet. The men agreed to eat less of most foods but did not need to change their food habits to any great extent. They cut down the sugar they ate by nearly two-thirds, they reduced the alcohol they drank by half, and their fat intake by one-third. Instead of eating over 3,100 calories a day, they ate only 1,600 calories until they had lost about 8 kg in weight and then went on a maintenance diet of about 2,300 calories.

It took the men an average of four months to lose the 8 kg, and then they continued on their maintenance diet for a further ten months without gaining or losing weight. On their maintenance diet, the men felt well and were as active as when they had eaten 25 per cent more calories.

What is relevant, and important, was Professor Blacket's finding that the blood levels of both cholesterol and triglycerides fell. The blood level of cholesterol fell by 10 per cent and that of triglycerides by 50 per cent to levels generally considered normal. The men achieved this by diet alone, without the use of drugs, which are often given to reduce high blood triglyceride and cholesterol levels.

The lesson of this investigation is clear. By over-eating, particularly by eating too many carbohydrate-rich foods and too many fatty foods, many of us in the affluent world are increasing our chance of a heart attack. That is the bad news.

The good news is that if we avoid over-eating—especially by cutting down the amount of sugar, alcohol, refined carbohydrate, and fat that we eat throughout our lives, but without markedly changing our food habits, we can avoid raising our blood levels of cholesterol and of triglycerides, which in some way may act as a trigger for a heart attack.

Perhaps as important, for those of us who are found to have high blood levels of triglycerides, is the finding that weight reduction alone, by diet, will reduce the high levels and will probably reduce our chance of having a heart attack.

Obesity is also associated with high blood pressure, which in turn is a factor in heart disease. An investigation in the U.S.A., involving more than one million people, has shown that men and women who were overweight, were at least twice as likely to have high blood pressure compared with people whose weight was normal. The research team also found that the higher the blood pressure, the greater was the likelihood the person would be overweight. It is clear from this that if a person avoided becoming fat, he or she would reduce the chance of developing high blood pressure and, indirectly, the chance of a heart attack.

The case against hypertension

Hypertension, or high blood pressure, is undoubtedly an accelerating factor in heart disease. For example, Professor Morris of London who has been studying this problem has recorded that among a group of middle-aged London bus drivers, who were studied for ten years, the higher the initial blood pressure, the greater the risk of developing coronary heart disease. In the U.S.A. a similar investigation showed the same result and it also showed that by reducing the high blood pressure a substantial reduction in heart attacks, strokes, and heart failure was obtained. 'Now', writes Professor Morris, 'moderate and severe hypertension can be lowered by today's potent and fairly well tolerated medicines.' But of course, you can't reduce the blood pressure until you find those people in the community who have a high blood pressure, and offer them treatment.

The test, as many people know, is really quite simple. In 1905, a Russian physician, Korotkoff, discovered that if a pressure cuff was applied to the upper arm, the blood pressure could be measured by listening to the sounds with a stethoscope over the artery in the fold of the elbow. With each heart-beat the blood pressure rises to a peak. This is called the systolic pressure. In between heart-beats the pressure falls to a lower level. This is called the diastolic pressure. By pumping up the cuff so that no blood flows through the artery and then releasing the air slowly, the blood flows in squirts and 'thumps' loudly on the artery wall which the doctor can hear through his stethoscope. This is the systolic pressure. As the cuff empties the character of the thumps changes and becomes soft. The change in sound identifies the diastolic pressure. Your blood pressure varies throughout the day and responds to all kinds of stress or emotion, when it tends to rise. During sleep it is at its lowest. The temporary rises are normal and natural, but the doctor tries to take a resting pressure. High blood pressure—hypertension—is diagnosed when the blood pressure is constantly above a certain level. In adults this level is usually said to be 150 mm of mercury for the systolic pressure, and 95 mm of mercury for the diastolic pressure. About one person in every ten over the age of 30 has a blood pressure above this level, and this individual is at increased risk of having a heart attack or a stroke when older. The risk is doubled if the diastolic blood pressure remains persistently above 110 mm of mercury. Not every person with a high blood pressure needs drugs. For many, weight reductions, regular exercise, the reduction of stress, and giving up smoking may be all that are needed. For others drugs will be required.

It will be apparent to those of you who have followed the confused and confusing epidemiological and experimental findings so far, that coronary heart disease is not caused by a single factor. Current opinion believes that it is the result of a constellation of factors, some of which may operate from birth, but most of which are aggravated by the way of life in the Western world. Coronary heart disease is a disease of an affluent overfed society. Several risk factors in our way of life tend to bring on heart attacks prematurely. The order of importance is in dispute, but the evidence I have presented suggests that a sequence may occur. Speculatively, the sequence goes like this:

If an individual eats excessive quantities of fats, especially saturated 'animal' fats, and perhaps of refined carbohydrates, particularly sugar, from early childhood, he is at greater risk of having a heart attack than an individual in a less sophisticated, and less overfed society. The fats, in susceptible people, lead to high levels of cholesterol in the blood which may eventually be a factor in atherosclerosis and heart disease. The excessive consumption of sugar and other refined carbohydrates has several consequences. They raise the blood triglyceride levels, and increase the stickiness of blood platelets. This encourages blood to clot and may be a factor in heart disease. The intake of more carbohydrates (especially sugar) and fats than are needed for energy constitutes 'empty calories' which are accumulated as body fat, and which result in obesity. Obese persons are more likely to develop diabetes, as are people who eat excessive quantities of sugar and refined carbohydrates over many years. Diabetes in association with obesity increases the risk of coronary heart disease. Obesity also predisposes an individual to high blood pressure, which in turn seems to be another factor in heart disease. In both men and women under the age of 40, cigarette smoking seems to play a more important role than high blood pressure. After the age of 50 the emphasis changes, and high blood pressure increases the risk of heart disease more than cigarette smoking. The place of exercise in the prevention of heart disease is unclear. It certainly helps to reduce obesity, but in sudden, unaccustomed bursts, exercise may be lethal. After a heart attack, regular, sensible exercise becomes increasingly important.

If the individual is tense, competitive, anxious, impatient, and unrelaxed, he is likely to eat (or drink) 'empty calories' excessively, he is likely to exercise fiercely or not at all, and he is likely to smoke heavily. Unless he can, in the words of St Matthew, 'change his foolish ways', he is asking for a heart attack. And he will probably get one!

Studies have been carried out, especially in the U.S.A., to see what the combined effect of the major risk factors is. In two large studies, involving over 10,000 men aged 40–59, who, when first examined, had no evidence of coronary heart disease, the factors of high serum cholesterol, high blood pressure, and cigarette smoking were examined. In these investigations, a high serum cholesterol was one of 250 mg per 100 ml serum or more; a high blood pressure was a diastolic reading of 90 mm of mercury or more; and cigarette smoking meant 10 or more cigarettes a day. The men were followed for 12 years. If none of the three risk factors were present at the beginning of the study, only 20 in every 1,000 men had a heart attack; if one was present, the risk of a heart attack doubled; if two were present, it doubled again; and if all three were present, the risk was eight times higher than that of the men who had none of the risk factors.

The evidence indicates that the risk factors are important; and with this knowledge it is possible to reduce the risk of a person developing coronary heart disease if he is prepared to alter his life-style and to modify his eating habits. It is not easy to persuade people to change their life-style, although there are hopeful signs as people become increasingly ecologically conscious, and reject excessive consumerism. The most sensible approach is for us to stop smoking and for us all to alter the character of our diet, so that we avoid the excessive consumption of saturated fat and sugar which is so much a part of our present dietary habits.

If too much fat in the blood—hyperlipidaemia—and excessive consumption of refined sugar are so deadly, when do they begin to have an effect? Increasing evidence, some of which I reported earlier, indicates that the process begins very early in life. Information from Australia, Germany, and the U.S.A. indicates that in the three countries, hyperlipidaemia is found in a significant number of infants by the age of one, and that by early adolescence one child in ten has a blood cholesterol over the 'ideal' upper limit of 220 mg per 100 ml of blood. By the age of 30, three men out of every four have a blood cholesterol level above the 'ideal'.

A blood cholesterol of 260 mg per 100 ml is considered by many cardiologists to indicate a high risk that the person will have a heart attack within 10 years. Of course this 'cut-off' figure is merely a statistic: about one man in every three who develops coronary heart disease has a blood cholesterol of under 260. And unfortunately the physician cannot tell which individual, in either group, is going to have a heart attack. He can only advise people of the risk.*

Nutritionists interested in heart disease are convinced that if the dietary habits of the individuals were changed, preferably from early childhood, the risk of heart disease would diminish. Unfortunately food habits are formed very early in childhood and are a doubtfully beneficial legacy from the parents, especially the mother. Once these habits have been imprinted on the brain, they are difficult to change and any attempt to do so is considered a threat to the individual's personal freedom, and an affront to his individuality.

Yet it is clear to the unbiased person that changes in our food habits have occurred over the years, and are occurring with increasing frequency since radio, and particularly television, have become so popular. The advertisers and the persuaders on the media manipulate our minds and alter our food habits, usually adversely. We can no longer consume, or wish to consume, peasant foods—cereals, breads made from unrefined flour, fruits, and vegetables, eating only occasional feasts of fatty meat—without being considered eccentric.

Instead, for many citizens of the rich nations every day is a feasting day. We tend, when we can afford it, to buy the fatter cuts of meat, which seem more tender. We enjoy eating cakes and biscuits, which have 'hidden' fat and sugar, and our desires are reinforced by astute advertising which links cake-baking with home-making. We reward our children for good behaviour by giving them sucrose-based sweets and chocolates, and television commercials stress their 'fun' value. We, and our children, swallow large quantites of sucrose-laden soft drinks. Ice-

---

* It is possible that as we learn more about the 'protective' nature of high-density lipid cholesterol, and the harmful nature of low-density lipid cholesterol, the doctor's advice may be more precise.

cream, based on coconut-oil, which has a very high sugar and saturated fat content, has become everybody's favourite. In England, for example, the gross consumption of ice-cream rose by 60-fold to over 60 million gallons a year in the 50 years between 1920 and 1970.

Breakfast cereals are now the usual way of starting the day. The craze, like many other crazes, started in the U.S.A. but has spread to Europe and other developed parts of the world. Breakfast cereals, it has to be admitted, are convenient. No cooking is required. All you have to do is to open the package and see the golden-glowing crispy flakes waiting for you to eat them. Open the package (it's so easy!) and pour out your bowl of crackling, tingling, zinging, popping, sugary, tasty flakes or puffs, add more sugar and some milk, and that's breakfast! But for what you get, they are overpriced, and poor value for money. Moreover, much of the advertising is misleading. An average breakfast portion of the common breakfast cereals weighs about 30 g (1 oz). Thirty grammes of cereal provides more empty calories than the same amount of wholemeal bread (because of added sugar) but fewer nutrients (calcium, iron, and vitamins of the B complex) and it costs between 2 and 5 times as much. As Dr Mann has written, 'Only the soap and cosmetic industries, promoting necessities and dreams, spend a larger fraction of income on advertising.' The promoters attempt to sell their products as 'low-calorie, low-fat' cereals to overweight adults with one hand, and with the other hand they sell the same products to undernourished children!

If there is to be a concerted attack on a disease which each year kills so many people, many people must be involved. Farmers and manufacturers must be persuaded to change their methods of production. Mothers, and more particularly potential mothers, must be given education in school in nutrition, diet, food selection, and preparation. And this education should be given to potential fathers—the boys—as well. One significant factor in producing bad food habits in schools is the school tuck-shop. In Australia, as in the U.S.A., this is often run by motivated concerned parents, and the profits raised help to run the school. Most tuck-shops sell the wrong foods, and by doing so reinforce poor eating habits. The persuasive manipulators of the media must be prevented from advertising food products in a misleading way, and must show responsibility in what they advertise.

The steps needed to change dietary habits were delineated in the U.S.A. in detail by the Inter-Society Commission on Heart Resources in 1970. Many authorities feel that some of their recommendations are invalid since their greatest concern was with saturated fats, and insufficient attention was paid to the consumption of refined carbohydrates. The recommendations are worth recording, however, because they represent the considered view of a large number of concerned biological scientists. I have to admit that, at present, we have no knowledge whether dietary measures, adhered to over the years, will actually prolong life and prevent heart attacks, but with the weight of evidence implicating our present eating habits in coronary heart disease, it would be prudent to accept that they might.

There is debate about the steps required to alter the dietary habits of a population. The process is difficult, for, as I have pointed out, dietary habits are imprinted on the human brain in early childhood and are difficult to dislodge. The Department of Health and Social Welfare in Britain, the Inter-Society Commission on Heart Disease in the U.S.A., the Scandinavian Medical Board, and the National Heart Foundations of Australia and New Zealand, among others, have made substantially similar recommendations. These recommendations require responsibility on the part of primary producers of foods, food manufacturers, and advertisers, and in this there may well be conflict as private profit diverges from the public good. They require a degree of education, and acceptance of dietary change by the consumer, although contrary to common belief the modifications to the diet of affluent, overfed, Western man can be made without a major dislocation of his eating habits.

The relative weight given to the recommendations, and the particular ones most stressed, differs in the various reports, but the key points remain the same. The points given here are listed in order of importance.

● A comprehensive and sustained public and professional nutrition education programme should be developed. In the

words of the American Inter-Society Commission, the programme should especially be directed 'towards developing
effective instructional programmes in educational curricula at
all levels, so that succeeding generations should have the
advantage of this knowledge from primary school'. Since children today are so influenced by the media, particularly television, new methods of education in nutrition need to be
developed, and time given in primary school, secondary school
and, for the minority, in tertiary educational institutions, for a
continuing programme. In adult life this needs to be reinforced
by the use of the most popular radio and television programmes
(which appear to be continuing drama series and personality
shows) to propagate good eating habits in an indirect, but
arresting way. The potentially beneficial role of women's
magazines should be utilized. The current emphasis in an
inordinate number of feature articles devoted (perhaps the
wrong word!) to making 'attractive' meals which are rich in fats
and refined sugars might be changed to conform with the
following suggestions.

● An educated, informed consumer has a right to know what he
is buying in the supermarket or corner shop. To this end the
packaging and labelling of foods, particularly manufactured
foods, needs more effective regulation to ensure that precise
labelling and definition of the foods is obtained. The consumer
has the right to know exactly what is contained in the food, and
in understandable amounts. In this respect recent regulations in
Britain are a good example of what may be done with little
distress, except to the dishonest manufacturer.

● There should be a considerable reduction in the saturated fat
content, the cholesterol content, and the refined sugar content
of baked goods, pastries, cakes, biscuits, etc., and consumers
should be encouraged to avoid these foods except on special
occasions. This need not change the taste of the food to any
great degree.

● A campaign should start to promote the use of fats and oils
which are low in saturated fat for cooking, shortenings, table
spreads, and salad dressings. This means that olive oil or

polyunsaturated oils should be used for cooking in preference to animal fats, including cooking margarines, which are based on animal fat or coconut oil. It means that individuals should eat less butter, and more polyunsaturated margarine, but it need not mean the total elimination of butter.

● Fatty meats are those in which the meat is 'marbled'. Usually such meat comes from animals reared in 'feed-lots'. The fat content of free-range animals is much lower. Much fatty meat is used in the manufacture of meat products, such as sausages, hamburgers, hot dogs, and other processed meat. Unfortunately, as far as your health is concerned, fat animals give the meat farmer a higher financial return, and many people have been conditioned to want 'marbled meat'.

Education is needed to induce people to reduce the amount of fatty meat products they eat and perhaps government action is also needed to increase the financial return to farmers whose beasts are reared free-range.

● Technological advances in the breeding of cows yielding milk with a reduced saturated fat and cholesterol content should be encouraged, so that both milk products and cheese of reduced saturated fat content are developed. This does not mean that milk and cheese should be avoided; these products have high nutritional qualities; it is the quantity eaten that needs to be considered.

● The encouragement of the consumption of refined sugar in drinks, and more particularly in sweets, cakes, and cooking should be reversed, as should the deceptive advertising of glucose for energy. The habit of rewarding children for good behaviour by giving them a sweet or a chocolate should be changed, since the early acquisition of a sweet tooth—and it is an acquired, not an inborn, characteristic—can, over the years, be lethal to some people. Ice-cream, which has acquired a status symbol, should only be permitted to be manufactured if based on polyunsaturated oil, with a limited sugar content. Coconut oil as a base for ice-cream manufacture should be banned. An effort should be made to change from eating expensive breakfast cereals to wholemeal bread, or to replace cereals with fruit.

What about you? Can you modify your diet to reduce your chances of having a heart attack? In 1974, a United States Select Senate Committee on Nutritional and Human Needs suggested six dietary goals. These are:

1. Increase the proportion of carbohydrate you eat, so that it makes up between 55 and 60 per cent of your calorie intake. Make sure that the increase is in the form of complex carbohydrates or starchy foods such as you obtain from whole grain, vegetables, and fruit.

2. Reduce your intake of refined sugar to 15 per cent of your calories. And don't forget that most of the sugar you eat is hidden in soft drinks, ice-cream, and confectionery.

3. Eat fewer fats; cut down your fats to 30 per cent of your calorie intake.

4. Reduce your intake of saturated fats to one third of your fat consumption.

5. Try to keep your daily cholesterol intake to about 300 mg a day.

6. Reduce the quantity of salt you eat to 3 g a day or less.

These goals can be put in the form of practical hints. Thus, to reduce your risk of coronary heart disease you should:

● Eat less sugar and fewer cakes, pastries, and biscuits. Instead, eat more wholemeal bread, vegetables, and any kind of fruit you enjoy.

● Eat less butter—or spread it more thinly. Don't eat too much cream: keep it for special occasions.

● Eat less fatty meat, and more fish or poultry. Choose lean meat: trim off visible fat. Grill it rather than fry it.

● Eat no more than one egg a day.

• Eat liver, kidneys, or shellfish no more than once a week.

• Use sunflower or olive oil rather than lard or hard margarine in cooking.

• Ask to have your serum cholesterol and triglycerides measured if either of your parents or any brother or sister had a heart attack before the age of 50; or if you have two or more risk factors (obesity, heavy cigarette smoking, or diabetes).

• Find out what kind of exercise you enjoy doing and do as much of it as you can.

• Don't smoke tobacco, but if you must, choose a pipe or a cigar and try not to inhale.

At the beginning of this chapter I pointed out that in the past decade deaths from coronary heart disease have declined, particularly among the 45–64 age groups, in all Western nations.

The reasons are not yet clear. Some deaths have undoubtedly been prevented by the development of intensive coronary care units in hospitals but, as only 70 per cent of those who have a heart attack reach hospital alive, this can only be part of the story.

The evidence points to the fact that more people are heeding the warnings about smoking and about having their blood pressure checked regularly and, if it is high, receiving treatment. At the same time, more people are changing their dietary habits. They are eating less saturated fat, less sugar, and fewer dairy products. They are eating more wholemeal bread, more vegetable fats, and fewer calories. These dietary changes may be the main reason for the beginning of the control of coronary heart disease.

Are you going to eat sensibly and help to avoid a heart attack? While you are thinking about your diet, don't light up a cigarette! Smoking not only causes lung cancer in susceptible people, but it contributes to heart disease and possibly other diseases as well. It is a serious health hazard.

9

Dietary crazes and crazy diets

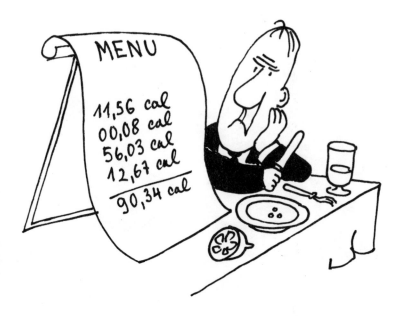

'Any literate person in a developed country has access to virtually unlimited advice on how to lose weight, and much of this advice is misleading. . . . There is probably no other field of medicine in which commercial pressures operate so directly against rational treatment.'   *J. S. Garrow, 1974.*

It is a sad paradox that, with the increasing availability of education and a wider range of information, mankind still persists in believing in magical remedies to avoid, or to cure, many diseases of modern civilization. Many people remain convinced that a copper bangle worn on the wrist will alleviate rheumatism; thousands, in desperation, seek worthless 'cancer cures', often at incapacitating expense. Similarly, millions consume large quantities of unnecessary vitamin and mineral supplements every day, which pass through their bodies unchanged, only to enrich the sewage.

In no area of health do magical remedies play a greater part than in the control of obesity. In 1979 a survey of a number of women's magazines in the U.S.A., Britain, and Australia showed that on average a new diet, claimed to be highly effective, was published in every third issue, only to be superseded by a diet claimed to be even more effective in the next issue but two. The desire of people in affluent countries to lose weight painlessly, quickly, and with as little disturbance to their way of life as possible, is the basis for the multiplicity of diets. Faith persuades them that the new diet will enable them to achieve this objective.

The modern obsession with dieting is also very profitable. Books about diet, if well publicized and promoted, sell millions of copies, especially in the U.S.A. Food fads and cults attract millions of people, who part with their money for the dubious, and usually temporary, satisfaction of 'feeling better'.

Food provides energy, and in an isolated system—such as a human being—energy follows the first law of thermodynamics: 'The energy in an isolated system is constant: any exchange of energy between a system and its surroundings must occur with the creation or destruction of energy.' If more energy is absorbed than is lost, weight gain is inevitable, and diets which claim that a method providing unlimited calories can simultaneously lead to weight loss are false.

Many published diets are essentially planned malnutrition; some are dangerous.

In the past 20 years, such diets have been published at about four-yearly intervals, mainly in the U.S.A. These diets have certain common features. First, the author insists that the diet shall have a low or very low carbohydrate content. Second, that the dieter does not need to restrict his total calorie intake. In other words, he may eat as much protein and fat as he likes, provided he avoids all or nearly all carbohydrate. The obvious attraction of such a diet in our affluent society is that you don't have to omit too many of the 'good things' you enjoy eating. These 'good things' are usually high in protein or high in fat or both.

The first diet in this century which confidently said that you could eat fat and get thin was introduced by Dr Alfred Pennington in 1953. He believed that fat people are fat because their metabolism quickly turned almost all the carbohydrate they ate into fat. He argued from this that if you cut out carbohydrate, almost completely, you could eat as much fat and protein as you liked and you would lose weight. But you should eat fat and protein in a ratio of 1 to 3. In other words you had to eat fat meat.

About eight years later, in 1961, the Pennington 'principle' was elaborated on by Dr Herman Taller in a book called *Calories Don't Count*. He believed that by eating lots of the right fats (mainly polyunsaturated fats) you set in motion a process which started you not only burning up the fat you ate but also burned up all the fats you had accumulated over the years in your adipose tissues. His lineal successor is Dr Robert Atkins, whose currently popular 'revolutionary' diet (which is neither new nor revolutionary) will be discussed later.

The fact that the theory was contrary to the first law of thermodynamics was contradicted by the 'evidence' of satisfied clients. And there were many. Dieting had become big business.

Several other diets followed which purported to let you eat what you like (so long as you didn't eat any carbohydrate) and let you drink what you liked. One such diet was published in 1964 by two authors (actually it was one writer who chose to use two pseudonyms) under the catchy title of *The Drinking Man's Diet*.

Then, in 1967 a new diet was announced by Dr Stillman. He agreed that calories did not need to be limited and that carbohydrate needed to be nearly eliminated, but he also discouraged you from eating fats. He said that the diet should be rich in protein (which in some way would melt away your store of adipose tissue), low in fats and very low in carbohydrates. Writing in collaboration with a journalist called Samm Baker, Dr Stillman's diet was published as *The Doctor's Quick Weight Loss Diet*. On this diet he allowed you to eat unlimited quantities of lean meat (with all the fat trimmed off); chicken and turkey (with all the skin removed); lean fish and any form of shellfish; eggs and cottage cheese or other cheese made from skimmed milk; but no carbohydrate or fruit. In addition, presumably to 'flush the kidneys', the dieter had to drink at least eight glasses of water a day. Dr Stillman's book has sold 10 million copies, and in its revised form apparently goes on selling.

Before these diets can be criticized, two points have to be made. First, the diets must work for some people for some time. Second, that they cannot be very successful as, after a period of about three years, they fade into relative obscurity, to be replaced by a revised version written in more racy language.

The truth is that although the diets appear to permit unlimited quantities of fat and protein, the dieter actually eats very little more than when he was not dieting. The diets, in effect, are low or no-carbohydrate diets *and* low calorie diets. Calories do count, and the first law of thermodynamics remains valid.

In 1974 a team of researchers led by Dr Rickman investigated twelve overweight people eating Dr Stillman's diet. They found that despite the opportunity to eat as much fat and protein as they wished, the twelve ate remarkably similarly amounts. Their average protein intake increased to 160 g compared with the 100 g eaten by Americans not on a diet. Their fat intake dropped to 73 g compared with the 115 g eaten by an average American, and, of course, their carbohydrate intake was very low indeed. This had the effect of reducing their average calorie intake from about 2,500 a day to about 1,300 calories a day. So of course they lost weight. In the first week of the diet, they lost far more weight than people on a 'balanced' low-calorie diet. In a balanced low-calorie diet, the carbohydrate component is never less than 50 g a day. Dr Stillman had stated in his book that this weight loss would occur: he had said that on his diet a person could lose '5–15 pounds per week'. The team confirmed that in the first two weeks of the diet a considerable loss of weight occurred, but they also found that this weight loss was very transient, and concluded that it was mainly loss of body water due to the severe restriction of carbohydrate (and, I would add, was probably the loss of most of the glycogen–water pool).

The loss of water also explains Dr Stillman's insistence that those people on his diet should drink at least eight glasses of water each day. If they did not, they would become dehydrated. In fact, most of the dieters complained of being easily fatigued, of lassitude, of mild nausea, and of occasional diarrhoea, and all found it difficult to stick to the diet and do their normal daily activities. Dr Rickman concluded, 'There seems very little reason for recommending the Stillman diet.' 'A diet low in calories', he said, 'would be far more likely to cause more lasting weight loss and would not bring about the unpleasant side effects which our subjects experienced.'

Support for this view comes from Dr Stillman himself, who in 1974 wrote another book which he has called *Dr. Stillman's 14-Day Shape-Up Program*. In this book he urges you to eat a high-protein, low-fat, *moderate* carbohydrate diet. Most nutritionists agree that a diet, however restrictive, should provide at least 50 g of carbohydrate a day if serious metabolic upsets are to be avoided. Dr Stillman now appears to recognize that some carbohydrate is desirable and his new diet provides at least 25 g of carbohydrate, which, although not enough, is in the right direction. His reported reason for the change was a social one, not a medical one: he found that a high proportion of those using his original diet cheated and ate some carbohydrate. Despite this change, neither of Dr Stillman's diets provide good nutrition, although he claims they do, and, in his latest book has made a vigorous attack on Dr Atkins' diet, which he claims is based on fallacy rather than fact and is not effective. While much doubt exists, as you will see, about Dr Atkins' diet, Dr Stillman's diet is not without its critics. For example, Philip White, spokesman for the American Medical Association's Council on Foods and Nutrition has written about Stillman's diet, 'It is essentially planned malnutrition. If you followed the diet as directed, you would actually lose protein from vital organs and other parts of the body. These losses could be quite devastating to somebody in poor health.'

In 1972 Dr Atkins, a fashionable New York physician, published his 'revolutionary diet'. Syndicated in women's magazines, it appeared in a hardback book carrying an evangelical dedication: 'to all diet revolutionaries who are not content merely to follow their own diet but who are dedicated to carrying the message of the diet revolution to the world which needs it'. These are stirring words indeed.

But on reading the book, it is neither as new nor as revolutionary as the author makes out. Dr Atkins' diet is a very low-carbohydrate, high-fat, moderate-protein diet, in contrast to Dr Stillman's very low- (now not so very low-) carbohydrate, low-fat, high-protein diet.

The book is written in easily-digested sections, interspersed with anecdotes of the diet's success amongst the notorious, the famous, and the successful. 'Imagine', says the blurb, 'losing weight with a diet that lets you have bacon and eggs for breakfast, heavy cream in your coffee, plenty of meat, and even salad *with* dressing for lunch and dinner.'

This appeal to the affluent and overfed, who crave for the 'goodies' of life but want to lose weight, met with instant success. How could it fail? But on reading Dr Atkins' book, grave doubts persist. He claims to have treated over 10,000 people successfully over a period of 10 years, yet he does not appear to have subjected his claims to any scientific study. He says that studies *should* be made, but has failed to make them himself. Despite this lack of scientific documentation, each chapter is written with confidence.

This confidence persists in a new book he has written (in collaboration with a medical journalist) *Dr. Atkins' Superenergy Diet*. In this he has discarded some of the more dubious beliefs he advanced in his first book. But in both books Dr Atkins makes certain claims which are disputed by most nutritionists. He claims that if you reduce your carbohydrate intake to a very low level, a substance called the 'Fat Mobilizing Hormone' is released. This hormone converts your body fat into carbohydrate, which is then converted into energy. No such hormone has been discovered, and biochemists have found that fat is not easily converted into carbohydrate. In the absence of carbohydrate in the diet, the breakdown of fat is incomplete, and acids accumulate, which are disposed of as 'ketones'. Dr Atkins is especially fond of ketones and attributes mystical values to them. He firmly asserts that on his diet they 'sneak hundreds of calories out of your body every day'. They don't. Two medical scientists, Dr Azar and Dr Bloom, measured the amount of ketones lost in the type of diet recommended by Dr Atkins and found that the quantity varied between 0.5 g and 10 g a day. A gramme of ketone excreted, carries about 4.5 kcals (about 20 kilojoules) of energy, so the greatest possible loss of calories due to ketones in his diet is about 50 kcals (200 kilojoules) a day, far less than the 'hundreds' he claims are lost.

Another claim by Dr Atkins is that many people who complain of lassitude, depression, and irritability have a low blood sugar, due to an 'excessive release of insulin'. Low blood sugar, or hypoglycaemia, he says, 'is unsuspected and undiagnosed to an extent without parallel in medicine'. This is not true. Concerned that many people might be deceived into believing that their tiredness, and feeling 'off-colour' might be due to hypoglycaemia, three major organizations, the American Diabetic Association, the Endocrine Society, and the American Medical Association, issued a joint statement in 1973. In this they wrote:

> Hypoglycaemia, means a low level of blood sugar. When it occurs, it is often attended by symptoms of sweating, shakiness, trembling, anxiety, fast heart action, headache, hunger sensations, brief feelings of weakness, and occasionally, seizures and coma. However, the majority of people with these kinds of symptoms do not have hypoglycaemia; a great many patients with anxiety reactions present with similar symptoms. Furthermore, there is no good evidence that hypoglycaemia causes depression, chronic fatigue, allergies, nervous breakdowns, alcoholism, juvenile delinquency, childhood behaviour problems, drug addiction or inadequate sexual performance . . .

In spite of this statement, Dr Atkins persists in his belief that hypoglycaemia exists and is due to high blood levels of insulin, which his diet in some way reduces. He gives no evidence to support his belief.

Whilst eating his diet, Dr Atkins also recommends that you

consume more vitamins. He is not alone in this, and many popular nutritionists also believe that 'mega doses of vitamins' make you more healthy. None of them has produced objective evidence for their claim and, as I have written in Chapter 6, excessive doses of vitamins merely add vitamins to the sewage and profits to the manufacturers.

It would be unfair and foolish to say there is nothing good about Dr Atkins' diet. As with Dr Stillman's diet, most people on Dr Atkins' diet cut down their total fat and only increase moderately the protein in their daily food. Because the diet is monotonous (and because Dr Atkins permits it) they add some carbohydrate to their diet quickly. By the end of three weeks most people on his diet will be eating 40–60 g of carbohydrate, about 70 g of fat and 150 g of protein, giving a total of 1,400 calories. This low-calorie, low-carbohydrate diet will produce a steady weight loss.

Dr Atkins rejects the use of drugs to reduce appetite, and of diuretics, which get rid of water. These suggestions are sensible. He also makes the suggestion that you keep a record of the carbohydrates you eat over a period of a few days before starting his diet. For most of us that would be a salutory and surprising exercise. Salutory because it will make us think about our diet; surprising when we find out just how much carbohydrate we unknowingly eat.

To some extent Dr Atkins's diet books have been superseded. In 1978 a Dr Tarnower, in collaboration with Samm Baker (once again), wrote *The Scarsdale Medical Diet*. Like Dr Stillman's all-protein diet and Dr Atkins's all-protein-and-fat-diet, the Scarsdale Medical Diet permits you to eat what you want—as long as you eat less than you usually ate in the past, which is sensible, if you want to lose weight. Then in 1979 a new diet 'that will not fail you' has appeared, under the title of *The Fabulous Fructose Diet*. Dr Cooper, who devised the diet, claims that fructose squelches your appetite, although it contains exactly the same calories as sugar. There is no evidence that fructose has this property, but if you read Dr Cooper's diet carefully you will find that you are expected to eat less. The fructose is the gimmick, the sense is that you ingest fewer calories if you stick to the diet.

By the time this book is published, a new infallible diet will

probably be on the book-stalls, which in its turn will be superseded in a year or two. And so it goes on.

Most of the other writers who provide the public with diets which
purport to enable them to eat what they enjoy and continue to
lose weight, also recommend that the person eats large doses of
vitamins, and other 'natural' foods.

Until she died in 1975, Adelle Davis was generally considered
the high priestess of popular nutrition. Like many other nutritional experts, who are vocal on radio, visible on television, and
voluble in magazines, she was a vitamin advocate. No other
'health-through-nutrition' expert has done more than she has to
popularize the need for people to eat large quantities of vitamins.

Unfortunately, her most popular book *Let's Eat Right to Keep Fit*
contains a nutritional or medical error on average on every
page, according to the nutritionist Dr George Mann; as does her
other best-selling book *Let's Get Well*, according to Dr Rynear-
son, Emeritus Professor of Medicine at the Mayo Clinic.

Some of her claims about vitamins are deceptive and some are
potentially dangerous. The deceptive claims include, for
example, the claim that niacin (one of the vitamins of B group)
will prevent 'blue Mondays'; that inosital (another possible B
vitamin) will cure baldness; and that calcium is a good pain-
killer. The potentially damaging claims are more serious. She
suggests that vitamin A should be taken in large doses over a
period, and that vitamin E will cure muscular dystrophy. These
treatments, if followed, will damage, not cure. She also makes
the statement that pregnant women should not drink skimmed
milk 'because it might cause cataracts in their babies'. This
statement is not only false, but may cause distress and anxiety.

It is difficult for the ordinary reader of her books to know what
is sensible nutrition and what is deceptive or damaging. In spite
of this, the books continue to be very popular.

If Adelle Davis was the high priestess of popular nutrition,
Charlton Fredericks is her successor. Both use much of the same
material; both quote the same authorities; both have similar, but
not identical, beliefs; both mix sound nutritional advice with

outrageous speculation, unsupported by evidence. This mixture is shown in the book Charlton Fredericks co-authored with a journalist, Herbert Bailey. The book *Food Facts and Fallacies* is just that—a mixture of facts, fallacies, and fantasy.

The book does give some good nutritional advice. Charlton Fredericks recommends that Americans escape their addiction to sweet, refined carbohydrates, and sugar-laden drinks. He suggests that tooth decay will be reduced as much by avoiding sweets and lollies, as by adding fluoride to the water supply. He condemns starvation diets and correctly says that, 'A reducing diet should be a miniature of a normal diet, so framed that expansion of the size of the portions will permit the diet to be used *after* weight loss has been stopped.' He correctly points out that protein releases the same amount of calories per gramme as does sugar and starch. He condemns the use of hormones and continued expensive, excessive psychotherapy, drugs, and surgery in the treatment of obesity.

These nuggets of good nutritional sense are embedded in a matrix of medical and nutritional misinformation and speculation. Errors of fact occur rather frequently. As well as this, Charlton Fredericks refers to the hundreds, and often thousands, of patients he has studied. But nowhere in the book are there any references to his published work, or indeed to many of the 'experts' he names and quotes, so that it is impossible to determine the validity of most of the statements he makes.

Robert Atkins, Adelle Davis, Charlton Fredericks, and the others have an exuberant confidence in their beliefs and the skill to communicate those beliefs in direct, easily understood language. When heard on the radio, and seen on television, their warm personalities were, and are apparent. They seem concerned about people. By contrast, many medical experts are uncomfortable when heard on radio and seen on television. They appear distant and superior, they appear to be unable to communicate easily, hiding instead behind a screen of jargon. It is not difficult to guess to which group the public will listen.

As well as the ability to communicate with the reader, viewer, or listener, popular nutritionists, like Adelle Davis, were critical of people's food and habits, at a time when the medical profession was largely silent. Adelle Davis, for example, criticized the over-processed, over-refined American diet, diluted with soft drinks, imitation juices, candy bars and "quick-energy" cereals', which, she said, 'has little or no relationship to wholesomeness'. She added, 'food supplements may help, but food itself is far more important'. She attacked the habit of giving babies glucose-water and formula feeds (instead of breast-feeding), and of starting salt-containing solids very early in infancy, before paediatricians spoke out on these matters. She attacked the influence of custom, persuasive advertising, and the desire to conform to neighbours' social norms which establish and perpetuate a craving for sugar and sweets in children, when such views were considered to be 'food faddist'.

The interest of people in dieting to obtain or maintain a good figure and glowing health, is exploited by the editors of women's magazines who manage to include a new 'miraculous' or 'revolutionary' diet in their publications at regular intervals. These diets appear with such rapidity and are so transient in appeal that it is difficult to know whether to mention any, in what it is hoped is a serious book, or whether to ignore them all. Two or three deserve mention, if only because they reappear at intervals, only to disappear, quite rapidly, when superseded by the next miracle cure.

At intervals, the 'Swedish liquid diet' appears under one name or another. The idea behind this diet is that if you only drink a semi-synthetic mixture of substances such as dried milk, soya bean powder with a trace of sugar, a dollop of vitamins, and a slurp of minerals, you can be given a measured number of calories a day, which will not exceed about 1,000 calories. On this diet you will, of course, lose weight, and money— for the prepared mixture is not cheap. You will also be bored with your food, but if you persist for a week or two (about half the people trying the diet manage to do this), you will find that you do actually lose weight. You will look forward with anticipation to the day when you achieve your target of weight loss because on that day you can stop this monotonous diet, and eat foods which taste good and which you enjoy. Usually, on that day, you start eating the foods you ate before you started the liquid diet, and, of course, your weight increases, until it is back to what it was before you started dieting. The diet has failed because it has broken a principle of a good reducing diet, that is, that the diet should be sufficiently palatable and varied to prevent you getting bored with it, so that you can continue with it for months.

Liquid diets, which are usually high protein, low calorie, and very low carbohydrate diets, may be dangerous. At the last count in the U.S.A. 60 people had died from the effects of the diet. All those who had died had used the liquid diet as their sole source of energy for extended periods. Others, who have not died, have had serious reactions. The Federal Drug Authority in the U.S.A. has issued a warning that liquid protein diets should only be used under strict medical supervision, and then not as the sole or primary source of calories for weight reduction.

There is also the grapefruit diet which continues to enjoy bursts of quite unmerited popularity. The grapefruit diet consists of grapefruit supplemented by little more than bacon and eggs. The grapefruit juice in some miraculous way is supposed to dissolve fat, so you can eat as much bacon and as many eggs as you like, provided you eat the grapefruit. It is, of course, hogwash. Grapefruit juice has no miraculous fat-dissolving powers. However, a regular intake of grapefruit may so disturb your taste buds that you don't feel a craving for sweet foods, and in this way it would help you keep away from alcohol, sugars, and starches.

Another popular, and useless, slimming diet is based on hard-boiled eggs, which in some mystical way are supposed to consume more energy than they provide. Soft-boiled eggs won't do apparently. The eggs have to be hard-boiled! This is absolute rubbish. Eggs, whether hard-boiled, soft-boiled or raw, release more energy than is used up in absorbing them.

To add to the effect of the chosen diet, entrepreneurs have provided other products which are claimed to enable you to lose weight painlessly. These products include slimming pills, whose main ingredient is usually a laxative; weight-reducing garments, which in some miraculous way are meant to melt fat; and additives to baths which, as you lie soaking in the hot water, are presumed to be absorbed through your skin and eat up your fat like termites! Unfortunately, for the purchaser, the products are of no value: you lose your money and keep your fat.

The popular appeal of diets, judged by the frequency with which they appear in magazines and by the sales of books on nutrition, suggests that people are interested in what they eat, and its effect on health. This concern has lead many people to reject the processed, artificially flavoured, sugar-rich foods available at supermarkets and shops. They choose instead to eat wheat germ, raw broccoli, raw carrots, and yoghurt. They are called 'food faddists'. But are they? According to *Nutrition Action*,

> The true food faddists are those who start the day on Breakfast Squares, gulp down bottle after bottle of soda pop, and snack on candy and twinkles. . . . This diet—high in sugar, cholesterol and refined grains—is the prescription for illness; it can contribute to obesity, tooth decay, heart disease, intestinal cancer, and diabetes.

10

A sensible diet
for Mr, Ms, and Mrs

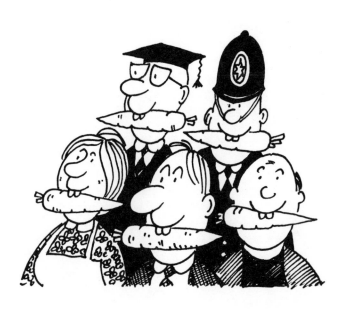

'Sir,
   I have followed your prescription as if my life depended upon it, and I have ascertained that during this month I have lost three pounds or a little more. But in order to reach this result I have been obliged to do such violence to all my tastes and all my habits—in a word I have suffered so much—that whilst giving you my best thanks for your kind directions I renounce any advantages from them and throw myself for the future entirely into the hands of Providence.'

Disappointed patient to his doctor, 1825.

'The twin objectives in devising a diet for the treatment of obesity are that it should be effective in removing excess fat and that it should become a permanent eating habit.'

John Yudkin, 1974.

This book should have made clear to you that the diet most of us eat today may be a major factor in a number of common diseases. If you want to avoid the chance of developing bowel diseases, obesity, coronary heart disease, diabetes, and others, you should modify your diet now. If you are obese, then you should start taking steps to reduce your weight.

If you are not overweight, you should consider eating a sensible diet. You can do this quite easily without altering your food habits radically. Here are some hints for sensible dieters:

• Eat more grains and beans, and more fruit and vegetables than you have done hitherto.

• Make sure that the cereal grains used in the food you eat are whole grains; cut down your 'refined carbohydrate' intake.

• If you can, eat wholemeal bread. The fibre in it assists the activity in your gut, and this in turn prevents constipation and reduces energy absorption from the food you eat. But it is not essential to choose wholemeal bread if you can't bear it.

• Reduce the amount of sugar you eat, and remember that sugar is hidden in many popular foods: cakes, pastries, biscuits, and shortenings.

• Reduce the amount of fatty meat you eat; replace it by lean meat, fish, or poultry. Don't fry your meat or your fish: grill it or casserole it. If you do fry fish, don't use any batter—it is mostly made up of carbohydrate.

• Reduce the amount of fat you eat, especially the hidden fat in cakes, shortenings, ice-cream, pastries, and biscuits.

• You can go on eating butter, but spread it thinly. You can eat eggs, if you enjoy them, but try to keep the number you eat to seven or less a week.

● Do eat some cheese and drink milk (either raw, in coffee or tea, or in foods) every day, to give you the calcium you need.

● Eat about 120 g (4 oz) or more of green leafy vegetables and some fresh fruit every day.

● If you eat a proper diet and are in good health you don't need vitamin or mineral supplements; save your money and buy fresh fruit or vegetables.

If you are overweight you have more of a problem, and it is only fair to state certain facts which have been discovered by scientists studying obesity. These are:

● In most published studies fewer than one-third of obese people lose more than 10 kg of weight, and only 10 per cent lose as much as 18 kg.

The implication of this finding is that it is better to prevent obesity than to have to go through the prolonged, discouraging, and uncomfortable process of getting rid of the extra fat and bringing your weight back to the normal range.

● The prevention of obesity should begin in infancy, since four out of every five fat babies become obese adults.

Much childhood obesity can be prevented if mothers follow certain suggestions:
First, breast-feed if possible rather than feeding your baby on artificial, formula cow's milk. Second, if you are unable to breast-feed, choose a low-sodium milk. Third, avoid introducing cereal semi-solid food supplements until your baby is at least four months old, and preferably six months old. Fourth, if you want to reward your child, or to soothe its hurt, it is better to avoid giving sweets and sugar-loaded drinks. Don't make your child a sugar addict! Instead choose fresh fruit juice, fruit, or wholemeal biscuits.
It is believed that a second dangerous time for laying the seeds of obesity occurs at puberty, that is between the ages of 11 and 14. If a child over-eats at this time, and particularly if the

child becomes a 'sugar-addict', the chances are that it will be more likely to become obese 10–20 years later.

School tuck-shops, which sell mainly 'junk' foods are run by devoted mothers, and by selling the food they do, the sweets, lollies, ice-cream, and all the other colourfully packaged sugar-loaded products, they are contributing to obesity.

Some of the children who have been overfed and who become obese may be unable to lose weight to any extent, when adult, unless they eat a starvation diet. Modest restriction of calorie intake fails to produce a weight loss. Dr Miller investigated a number of these diet-resistant obese people. He found that they had 'adapted' to use less energy for their needs than other obese people and they had more fat cells in their bodies. You can't identify which fat person is of this type, so that it is sensible to avoid infant and childhood obesity.

The remedy is in the hands of parents, and teachers. What are you doing about it?

● The only person who can treat your obesity is you—with a little help from your friends and advice from a nutritionist.

By itself a diet chart is useless, you have to be motivated to keep to the diet and to understand it. Your ability to keep to your diet requires motivation: it is all too easy to cheat—just a little. Motivation is stronger if you can share your experiences and obtain support from other people who are also trying to lose weight. That support needs to extend over the period of weeks or months when you eat the reducing diet with its limited calories. It is also a help to have support to keep you motivated to retain your new lower weight once you have shed the kilograms required to reach it!

This is where organizations like TOPS (Take Off Pounds Sensibly) and WWI (Weight Watchers International) are very helpful. They provide a form of group therapy to keep you motivated. The value of WWI in helping people to lose weight can be judged by a study made in Adelaide, Australia, where Dr Williams and Dr Duncan conducted an Obesity Clinic at the Royal Adelaide Hospital. They compared the weight loss of people attending their clinic (some of whom also received hunger-reducing drugs) with the weight loss of people who joined WWI. Dr Williams found that those who joined WWI lost more weight each week and remained longer at their lower weight than did those who attended his Obesity Clinic. This demonstrates the importance of motivation and the value for many people of organizations like WWI.

● If you want to lose weight you have to discipline yourself to eat less energy than you use up.

This means that you have to eat fewer calories than before, and if possible, exercise more.

● There is no magical instant cure for obesity.

Although it is fairly easy to lose between 3 and 6 kg of weight quickly, it is hard to prevent the relentless return of that weight unless you discipline yourself to go on eating fewer calories than you use up.

● Permanent weight loss is a slow process, whatever the purveyors of miraculous diets say.

No diet is miraculous. 'Wonder-diets' don't work, except briefly. But if you can manage to keep to a diet which provides you with 500–1,000 calories less than you need, you will burn up your stored fat at a rate of about 0.5–1.0 kg a week. Over six months that amounts to about 18 kg.

To obtain a clearer understanding of this important matter, it is necessary to recall the composition of the body of an average man who weighs about 72 kg (158 lb or 11 st 4 lb). Fifty kilograms of the total consists of water and minerals. Six kilograms of his weight is accounted for by the protein which makes up his muscles, and is intimately connected with all his vital organs, so that even in advanced starvation very little is available for energy. Less than 0.3 kg of his weight is due to carbohydrate, but the fatty tissues in his body weigh 12 kg. This fat is available for energy needs and if burned up completely would release about 90,000 calories.

Men weigh more than women as a rule. A typical obese,

middle-aged woman, whose height is 1.60 m (or 5ft 3 in) and who weighs 72 kg, is about 17 kg overweight, and most of this excess is due to fat she has made and stored over the years when she has eaten more energy in the form of food than she has used up. Mrs Smith, the typical woman, has read articles and is worried about being too fat. She would like to get back to her ideal weight of 55 kg (121 lb, or 8 st 9 lb). Each day she probably requires to expend about 2,000 calories of energy to meet the demands of her body and her work in the house. If she could manage to eat only 1,000 calories a day, it would take 125 days—over four months—before she exhausted her stored energy by burning up the fat she had laid down over the years. A diet of only 1,000 calories a day is very difficult to stick to, so it is more likely that she would choose a diet which provided 1,500 calories a day. On this diet, if she stuck to it exactly, she would burn up 500 calories of stored energy each day and it would take her 250 days—over eight months—for her weight to fall to the ideal! Mrs Smith has a real problem, for it is stupid to pretend that it is easy to lose 17 kg of weight and it is unlikely, whatever diet she decides upon that she will manage to do it in less than eight months.

As well as this, previously fat people who have managed to reduce their weight by dieting regain weight very quickly, compared with untreated fat people, if they start over-eating again. For this reason, Mrs Smith will have to exert very great willpower to achieve her weight loss and to keep to her lower weight. Doctors do not really treat obesity; they only help fat people to treat themselves.

● Even on a slimming, low-calorie diet, your weight may fluctuate. Don't be discouraged. If you keep unswervingly to your diet you will succeed in losing weight!

● Be sure that your chosen diet permits you to enjoy a social life. It is pointless to be a thin, antisocial, crotchety recluse—better to be fat, happy, and enjoying life. Becoming thin should not be made a penance, nor should the obese person be filled with guilt as well as fat. There are slimming diets which enable you to eat most of the foods habitually eaten by your family and to eat when you socialize with your friends.

• When on your diet do take more exercise—if you enjoy it. Don't exercise and hate it. You will compensate for your dislike by over-eating.

It is helpful if you go for a walk, or do something active, after a meal. There is evidence that this helps you lose weight rather more quickly than if you slump down in front of the television set as soon as you have finished eating. This is because exercise induces heat production and energy loss.

• Don't go on a 'crash diet' which provides less than 500 calories a day. Initially these diets do produce a more rapid weight loss, but after a while you will find you can't keep to the diet, and when you stop you usually over-eat. Oddly enough it has been found that on a crash diet you burn up lean body tissue (mostly protein) rather than fat—in fact you burn up no more of your fat stores on a 'crash diet' over a two-month period than if you chose and stuck to a 1,000 calorie diet.

Crash diets and crazy diets don't really help, despite what the magazines and your friends say. For a short while they seem to succeed, but sooner rather than later you find you can't keep to the diet and you over-eat. Back comes the fat—and you become discouraged!

• Choose a diet which is nutritious, and which is sufficiently varied and tasty to enable you to stick to it without getting bored or frustrated. As far as weight loss is concerned it doesn't matter too much what proportions of carbohydrates, protein, and fat you eat in your diet, so long as it is a low-calorie diet, and so long as it contains sufficient vitamins, minerals, and roughage (fibre) to keep you in good health. But make each meal attractive to look at, pleasant to smell, and good to taste, so that you learn to enjoy your diet.

• If you limit the 'fibre' in your food you may become consti-pated and be at risk of other unpleasant disorders. The remedy is easy: eat wholemeal bread in your ration and if you need to, take two dessertspoonfuls of coarse bran daily. It won't add to your carbohydrate or calorie intake, and it will help you to avoid the side-effects of a 'refined carbohydrate' diet, which are thought to include diverticular disease and haemorrhoids.

• Don't gorge by eating only one large meal a day. You will lose weight more quickly if you eat several small meals spread out over the day—and you will feel more normal if you do this. Don't miss breakfast and don't eat your last meal late at night. The reason for eating several small meals rather than a single large meal is that smaller meals eaten at shorter intervals induce a greater production of body heat, which is then dissipated into the surrounding air. Body heat is produced by using energy, and that is what you are trying to do—to use more energy than you ingest.

• Do try and eat your meals at approximately the same time each day. This has the psychological effect of helping you to control your feelings of hunger at times other than meal times.

• When you have a meal, eat slowly. When you have put food in your mouth don't add any more until your mouth is empty. If it helps, put down your knife, fork, or spoon while your mouth has food in it. And chew your food slowly so that you learn to taste and smell the food to the fullest extent. Psychologists believe that eating slowly and chewing meticulously teaches you to be satisfied with less food and to enjoy the smaller quantity more.

• Every fifteen mouthfuls, stop and put down your eating utensils for about half a minute. This strategy helps you to enjoy more the smaller amount of food you are permitted.

• Before you start eating, decide how much of which food you are going to put on your plate, and don't add more. Once you start eating it is too easy to say to yourself, 'I'll just have a little more.' You mustn't. 'Littles' add up to a lot and you will not control your eating. It often helps if you put your food on a smaller plate, so that the plate looks fuller! This will help you make do with less.

• As soon as you feel full, stop eating, no matter how much is still on your plate. Indeed, it may help you always to leave some food on your plate, and so break the habit of continuing to eat until all the food on your plate has gone, whether you need it or not.

● Once you feel full or finish your meal, leave the table (if you can do so without offending anybody). Staying at the table where there is food may break your resolve not to eat any more.

● Only go shopping for food when you have eaten. If you do your own shopping, or shop for the family, you may be tempted when you see the delicious-looking foods in the shops. You can resist the temptation to buy and eat these foods if you do three simple things. First, only go shopping after you have eaten. People react less to the sight of food when they are not hungry. Second, make out a list of foods you really need before you go shopping. Stick to the list. Don't be tempted by other foods. Third, when possible only buy foods which need more preparation than just opening the container. This will reduce the risk that you will 'just open a tin or a packet for a little snack'.

● Don't be 'conned' into choosing a complicated or expensive diet. You won't keep to it. Diets which insist that you only eat certain foods on certain days, and other foods only at certain times of the day, should be avoided. They are rubbish. Choose a diet which is no more expensive than your usual food. If you don't, someone will complain and you will become discouraged and stop eating your diet.

● Don't keep packets of sweets or chocolate in the house. If you get bored or unhappy you will be tempted to have a nibble. If they aren't there you can resist the temptation. If they are, you will be able to resist everything except the temptation.

● Before you start a slimming diet, you have to decide for yourself that you really want to lose weight. Unless you are convinced, you won't keep to your diet. And unless you keep to your diet you won't lose weight. It won't be quick. It will take weeks or months. But you will do it!

● Don't believe that drugs will help you—except, perhaps, in the first few weeks of your diet. During these weeks, hunger-suppressing drugs may help you to adjust to your slimming diet more easily. But remember all the hunger-suppressing drugs have some unpleasant side-effects, and they only suppress hunger for about 6–10 weeks at the most.

● A few people fail to lose weight despite dieting. Even on a diet that only provides 1,000 calories a day some chronically fat people are unable to lose a significant amount of weight. They don't put on weight, but they don't lose it as they had hoped they would. These people—most are women—have usually been fat since infancy. They have more fat cells in their bodies than other people, and they use up energy less efficiently. In other words they have adapted biologically to using fewer calories for their needs.

If you are one of these people and you have conscientiously kept to your diet for a period of months without losing weight, I am afraid you are going to remain fat. Don't put on any more weight, but don't feel guilty. Enjoy life!

It would make many fat people happy if it were possible to report that a drug had been developed which enabled them to become thin without having to go through the discipline and self-denial of dieting. Man seems to have an almost mystical faith in medicines, particularly if they appear to help him do something he finds uncomfortable or distasteful.

Because of this hope, fat people keep on seeking a drug which will make them lose weight painlessly, quickly, and without altering their diets. There is no such drug, but it is a fertile area for bogus theories, for cures recommended by relatives, and for unscrupulous and deceptive advertising.

Matters have not changed much since 80 years ago, when Dr Thomas Dutton wrote in his book *Obesity*, 'quite a host of quack nostrums are advertised . . . to say the least of them, they are altogether unscientific and in many cases positively injurious'. In Dr Dutton's day excruciating purges and strong salts were fashionable. Today diuretics, hormones, 'bulk fillers', and 'pep-pills' are popular. Most are used unscientifically, except in

rare and very special circumstances, and some may be positively injurious.

A diuretic is a drug which acts on the kidneys, preventing
water being reabsorbed into the body. The drugs are very useful
for patients in heart failure whose body is swollen with excessive water. The use of the drugs in treating obesity is quite
unjustified. Since about 60 per cent of your body weight consists of water (mostly bound in cells), it is true that a dramatic,
but transient, weight loss can be obtained by the misuse of
diuretics. But this is a most unwise therapy. Body weight will
fluctuate wildly. If it is down the hopeful slimmer will be
delighted, and will tell her friends she has found an easy cure
for obesity. But if she weighs herself regularly, she will sooner
or later find that despite her diet, her weight has increased and
she will be despondent. It will convince her that her diet is not
working, and that she is the kind of person who can never lose
the excess weight. The reason is that diuretics only get rid of
water from the body. A fat person is fat because he or she has
large fat stores which have to be used up before the desired
weight reduction is obtained. So don't ask for, recommend, or
use diuretics to treat your obesity.

Hormones, especially thyroid preparations, have been popular in recent years. Thyroid preparations, if given in dangerous
doses to a normal person, will raise his metabolic rate and will
increase his weight loss. But the improvement is short-lived and
the treatment is potentially dangerous, so there is no justification for taking thyroid tablets to lose weight, unless tests have
shown that you have a deficiency of the thyroid hormone produced in your body. This is quite uncommon. If you haven't, by
taking thyroid tablets you are merely substituting one disease—thyrotoxic thyroid disease, for another—obesity.

Another hormone, human chorionic gonadotrophin, or
HCG, given by injection at intervals has been claimed to lead to
weight reduction and is used by various 'fringe' doctors who
'specialize' in treating obesity. The basis of this treatment is the
belief that HCG injections dissolve body fat.

HCG was introduced in 1949 by Dr Simeons, an English
doctor then practising in Rome. He injected a small amount of
HCG (125 International Units) daily and combined this with a
500 calorie diet. The first course lasted at least 23 days, and,

naturally, the client lost weight. Dr Simeons claimed that HCG 'was in some way specifically concerned with the control of obesity', but he never determined the way in which it was effective. There is no scientific evidence that HCG has any effect on weight loss, states an American Medical Association report, after examining the evidence.

The HCG therapy works by putting the client on a 'crash' 500 calorie diet and this is not without danger. According to Dr Drenick, Professor of Medicine at the University of California, a 500 calorie diet can induce hair loss, dry scaly skin, and possibly ketosis.

The value of the HCG method lies not in the injections but in the client's mind (who believes that they will work) and in the fact that each day the client has to attend to receive an injection. At this visit the client receives the strong psychological support from a counsellor. In contrast, the potential danger of HCG plus a near-starvation diet is such that a diet can lead, in a few weeks, to malnutrition.

Of course, clients rarely remain on the diet long enough for this to happen. They become too hungry and usually increase their food intake to at least 1,000 calories a day.

In summary, HCG injections have no known effect on weight loss but may help a person to keep on a strict diet. They are an expensive and not really effective way of providing psychological support.

Obviously, if you can reduce a person's appetite, either by using a drug which acts on the appetite-controlling centre in the brain, or by filling the stomach with an inert substance, so that a feeling of repletion occurs, you will reduce your food intake. For a time, stomach 'bulk fillers' were popular. Usually made of methyl cellulose in the form of a biscuit, they were eaten an hour before a meal in an attempt to enable the person to resist food. The theory is that in the stomach they swell rapidly—like a sponge—by absorbing the stomach fluids—and so give the feeling of fullness. Recent research has shown that this belief is not exactly true. Bulk fillers swell relatively slowly and are unlikely to reach their full bulk before leaving the stomach, so that they act as laxatives rather than appetite suppressants. However, they are harmless and may help people who have a psychological need for 'drugs' to help them keep to their diets.

The true appetite-suppressing drugs are related chemically to 'pep-pills' or 'purple hearts'. These are the amphetamines which act directly on the appetite-controlling centre in the brain, diminishing the feeling of hunger or increasing the sensation of 'feeling full'. Amphetamines carry a serious danger of addiction and are no longer used, but some doctors recommend their newer derivatives, and other appetite-suppressing, or anorectic, drugs in the management of obesity.

Four drugs are currently used. Three of these are amphetamine derivatives and one is not. The amphetamine derivatives are diethylproprion (Tenuate, Tenuate Dospan), phentermine (Duromine), and fenfluramine (Ponderax). The drug which is not derived from amphetamines, but which the manufacturers claim suppresses appetite even better than amphetamine derivatives, is called mazindol (Sanorex).

Unfortunately, the drugs have side-effects which affect between 20 and 25 per cent of people. The side-effects are dryness of the mouth, irritability or depression, drowsiness by day or sleeplessness at night, and occasionally nausea or diarrhoea.

Careful research suggests that if the drugs are used, they are only effective in suppressing the appetite for six to ten weeks, but during this time they may help a fat person, who finds it difficult to stick to his low-calorie diet at the beginning of weight reduction courses, to do so. Unfortunately when the drugs are stopped the person's appetite tends to increase, just as it does if the drugs are continued for periods longer than ten weeks. If the drugs are used, they should only be taken on the advice of, and under supervision by, a doctor.

Two other substances not usually classed as drugs should be considered, since people on diets often ask about them. The first is alcohol, the second tobacco.

Alcohol is pleasant, it makes you feel good, and it does cause some heat loss as it makes your skin vessels dilate. However, alcoholic drinks contain calories, so you have to limit your alcohol intake as well as your food intake if your diet is to work.

Many people complain that when they stop smoking they put on weight. They are telling the truth, since cigarettes, particularly, reduce your appetite. However, cigarette smoking is a risk factor in heart disease, stomach ulcers and lung cancer, so it is best avoided—if you can!

Most people who have massive obesity—which means they are more than 50 kg above their 'ideal weight'—find that diet, even when supplemented by counselling, is ineffective to produce changes in eating behaviour. If the massive obesity is associated with life-shortening diseases, such as high blood pressure or gall-bladder disease, or with a disabling condition such as arthritis, surgery may be recommended. The operation involves 'by-passing' that part of the small intestine, the jejunum, from which most food is absorbed. The upper end of the jejunum is cut and is stitched to the lowest part of the small bowel. Weight loss occurs, first, because the person eats less after operation; second, because what is eaten is less well absorbed; third, because the person has a reduced desire to eat sweet foods. In the year after operation most people lose over 25 kg of weight and feel better, with greater self confidence and a higher self-esteem. They feel better because they look better!

Unfortunately the operation is not without danger. Five per cent of those operated on, die; either due to the operation or within the first year, and about one person in three develops disturbing complaints, including frequent bowel movements and even more frequent uncontrollable bouts of 'gas' and bursts of 'passing wind'. More worrying are reports that between 5 and 20 per cent of those who have 'bypass' surgery develop progressive liver damage, kidney stones, arthritis or bone disease.

In spite of articles which have appeared in women's magazines, surgery should only be used in very rare cases of really gross obesity which may reduce considerably the person's life expectancy, and when symptoms of breathlessness and severe backache make life disabling. Because of the complications and because the best results are obtained in hospitals which have a team of skilled surgeons, biochemists, psychiatrists and others working on the problem, anyone who is thinking about having the operation should be treated and followed-up after operation in such a hospital. Jejuno-ileal bypass is still experimental and much more has to be learnt before it can be recommended.

If you have managed to read this far without getting too depressed, you will have your reward! There are several slimming diets which meet the criteria of being no more expensive than normal diets, which are reasonably palatable and varied, which permit you to eat more or less what your family and friends eat, and which can be continued, without boredom, for as long as you wish. If you are obese, you may have to continue dieting all your life.

A slimming diet which appeals to me more than most is the one recommended by Professor John Yudkin in his book *This Slimming Business*. On this diet, which is a low-carbohydrate, low-calorie diet, you limit your carbohydrate intake to between 50 and 100 g a day, but you can eat as much protein and fat as you like. As Professor Yudkin points out, 'eating as much as you like' is not the same as 'eating a large amount'. In fact, people on his diet in general eat no more fat and only a little more protein than people who are not dieting normally eat. It is also necessary to point out that a low-carbohydrate diet is quite different from the 'no'-carbohydrate vitamin-supplemented diets so persuasively recommended by some 'experts', and discussed in Chapter 9. In Professor Yudkin's diet over 15 per cent of the energy is supplied by carbohydrate, and the dangers of ketosis and high blood cholesterol level are avoided.

A further advantage of the diet is that it is relatively simple to calculate what you may eat. You only have to know how much carbohydrate there is in those commonly eaten foods which contain carbohydrate. These you may remember are sugar, bread, confectionery, cakes, biscuits, soft drinks, alcohol, potatoes (and other root vegetables), rice, milk, and fruits. You don't have to bother about foods which have no carbohydrate. These include meats, fish, poultry, cheese, eggs, leafy vegetables, and butter.

Of course, you have to be sensible. You would be a fool if you stuffed yourself with non-carbohydrate foods. That would be irresponsible and, anyhow, your craziness wouldn't last long. You'd get bored! As well as this it is more sensible to grill your meat, fish, or poultry rather than fry it. But that isn't essential for the diet.

All in all, the low-carbohydrate, low-calorie diet has advantages over other diets and it seems to be sensible diet for those fat people who want to lose weight, or indeed for those people who tend to get fat and want to avoid doing so.

Full details of the diet are to be found in Professor Yudkin's book. He makes the point that his diet is neither new nor based on an extraordinary discovery about man's metabolic processes. The diet is not based on fallacy, but on scientific fact (perhaps slightly biased, some nutritionists would say, but on fact nevertheless).

The diet is low in carbohydrate. That means you have to discipline yourself to cut down—or to cut out—some of the foods to which you have become addicted over the years.

The first is sugar. Sugar is pure carbohydrate and contains nothing but energy. That is why it is said to contain 'empty calories', for it provides no nutrients to the body. Sugar just provides energy, but in our Western diet the energy needed is provided as easily and more nutritiously in other foods. So, out goes sugar, and that includes sweets, chocolates, cakes, and ice-cream!

In any addiction, withdrawal of your drug causes upsets. When you stop using sugar you may find that you crave to add it to your tea or coffee or to your breakfast cereal (if you eat one, and you probably should not!).

You can deal with this craving in one of two ways. Which you choose will depend on your personality. The first way is to stop at once. You stop using sugar in tea or coffee, you avoid using sugar on breakfast foods and you stop eating sweets, cakes, or chocolates. The second way is to be more gentle to yourself. If you habitually add three spoons of sugar to your cup of tea, cut it down to two, and then after a few days, to one. In other words, wean yourself gradually from your craving for sugar and sweet foods.

The second addiction you may have is to alcohol. Although alcohol is not strictly a carbohydrate it provides energy in the same way. And many of us enjoy a drink! Again, you can be very firm with yourself and drink soda water with a slice of lemon and, if you wish, a dash of angostura bitters in place of your favourite drink. Or if you are less strong, you can, if you wish, have 250 ml (10 oz) of beer, or 30 ml (1 oz) whisky, or 125 ml (5 oz) of a light wine a day. Each of these provides about 20 g equivalent of carbohydrate, or about 80 calories of energy. But you must not add bitter lemon or ginger-ale to your whisky, or drink either of these alone, as they contain a fair amount of sugar, whatever their taste. You can only have water or soda water which contain no calories.

Apart from these restrictions you should work out your own diet. You can either do this as Professor Yudkin suggests, using 'carbohydrate units' (one unit equals 5 g of carbohydrate) or you can calculate your carbohydrate intake in grams. If you choose to use grams you need to restrict your intake to between 50 and 100 g a day, depending on how much you are overweight, how quickly you want to get rid of the extra fat, and how strong your will-power is.

Since you are only calculating your carbohydrate intake you only have to worry about foods which contain significant amounts of carbohydrate. You can ignore, that means you can eat as much as you wish of, the following: meat, fish, eggs, cheese, butter (or margarine), green leafy vegetables, and most fruits. But you should not eat more than two or three slices of bread each day, and you should not eat cakes or pastries at all.

The attraction of this diet is that within certain limits you eat as much the same foods as the rest of your family, and so you don't feel outcast and different.

THE YUDKIN DIET
modified and simplified

You can eat as much of these foods as you like — but be sensible!

Meat	Butter
Fish	Cheese
Eggs	Green leafy vegetables

You can eat a limited amount of these foods:

Milk:	up to 600 ml (1 pint) a day.
Fresh fruit:	not more than two of the following a day: apples, oranges, grapefruit, pears, peaches; or one of the above and an average serving (about 120 g or 4 oz) of strawberries, raspberries, gooseberries, plums, blackberries, cherries, or grapes.

You must restrict these foods because they contain carbohydrate, although you can substitute one for the other:

Bread (preferably whole-meal)	Potato, average size
Oatmeal	Baked beans
Biscuits	Nuts
Cornflakes	

In a day you can have up to three slices of bread (depending on how quickly you want to lose weight) or the equivalent. Remember the calorie content of the following is about equal:
$1\frac{1}{2}$ slices of bread = 1 average potato = 3 small sweet biscuits = 1 average serving of oatmeal porridge, or cornflakes, or baked beans.

You must avoid these foods, as they are either completely or mostly carbohydrate:

Sugar (raw or refined)	Cakes and buns
Sweets and chocolates	Canned fruits
Jams and honey	Soft drinks (except soda
Pastries and puddings	water)

You should avoid alcoholic drinks, but if you can't, limit yourself to one of the following:

Beer	250 ml ($\frac{1}{2}$ pint)
Whisky	30 ml (1 measure)
Wine	125 ml (1 glass)

It may well be that while you are on a diet you are invited out to a dinner party. You don't have to be embarrassed, or embarrass your hostess, by toying with your food and leaving most of it on the plate. You just have to be sensible and enjoy yourself. You miss out the bread roll and the pudding unless it is a fresh fruit salad, and you limit the amount of alcohol you drink. You only take one potato, but you eat everything else. If you do exceed your daily quota of carbohydrates, well, it is a special occasion and it won't make much difference in the long run.

The diet Professor Yudkin suggests seems to meet the criteria a diet should have. It is nutritious, it is low in calories, it is relatively easy to understand and to follow, and it doesn't make you feel a freak, it avoids gimmicks, and you can stay on it for a long time, and most important of all, it works! These criteria seem to me to form the basis of a sensible diet for a sensible person.

But a diet will only work if you really want to lose weight and are prepared to understand and stick to the diet over a period of months.

In the end, it is up to you.

APPENDIX

The food we eat

By the time we become adults most of our body is composed of water. Over 60 per cent of our body weight is water, nearly all of which is held in the billions of cells which make up our body. Fat, unless we are obese, makes up between 11 and 18 per cent of body weight. Protein accounts for 15 to 20 per cent, minerals for 5 per cent, carbohydrate for less than 1 per cent, and there are also tiny, but vital traces of vitamins.

Fats

As you may remember from Chapter 1, the fat stored in your body is mainly held in your adipose tissues.

Careful scientific investigations have shown that about four-fifths of adipose tissue is composed of fat cells and the balance is made up mainly of water (20 per cent), with a little protein (2 per cent). This means that if you can calculate the amount of adipose tissue in your body, the amount of stored fat will be one-fifth less. This fat is available to be released to supply energy when your energy intake is inadequate for your current needs. Unfortunately the fat in your adipose tissues is released rather slowly, and you may need to obtain energy from your stores more rapidly.

You can do this because you have a second and equally important energy storage system in your muscles. In between the fibres which form your muscles the substance glycogen is stored, dissolved in water. Glycogen, combined intimately with water, makes up the 'glycogen–water pool'. In an average person the pool weighs between 4 and 6 kg. One to one and a half kilograms consists of glycogen, and the remaining 3–4½ kg consists of water. Each gram of glycogen, when mobilized, releases 4 calories of energy, but in the process the body loses 3 g of water. In starvation, when little or no energy is supplied to your body because little or no food is eaten, the first release of the energy you need comes from the glycogen–water pool. This means that in the first week of starvation, when you need at least 6,000 calories to keep your body working, you will lose between 4 and 6 kg of weight. Since most of this loss is water, the rapid weight loss is only transient, for when the starving person eats once again, the glycogen–water pool is remade and he regains most of the weight he lost. If the person now eats a diet providing fewer calories than he uses, the weight loss will continue, but only slowly, as now he will burn up fat stored in his adipose tissues.

The size of the glycogen–water pool is relatively constant in most people, but the adipose tissue stores vary very considerably, as we discussed in Chapter 1. To a large extent their size depends on the quantity and type of food you have eaten over the years, the amount of exercise (or lack of exercise) you have taken, but other factors, including genetic ones, play a part. It is interesting too, that your gender influences the size of your fat stores. Women, on average, have nearly twice as much fat stored in their bodies as men have.

Your fat stores are not an inert energy bank ready to release energy when you fail to obtain enough from your diet. On the contrary, the stores are dynamic.

Fat is constantly being deposited in the storage cells of the adipose tissues in the forms of drops of triglyceride, and is constantly being released from the storage cells in the form of fatty acids. The breakdown of the fatty acids then releases their stored energy.

Until recently, energy was measured in kilocalories (calories or kcals are the same thing). The definition of kilocalorie is a bit complex, but it is based on heat produced when a food is completely burned up in oxygen. A kilocalorie is defined as the amount of heat required to raise the temperature of a litre of water from 15°C to 16°C.

In 1970, after international consultation, scientists decided that this was an inappropriate measure of energy, and devised a new one, which they called a joule (J). This is the amount of energy expended when one kilogram is moved one metre by a force of one newton. This definition is even more complicated unless you are a student of physics, so in this book, the old-fashioned term calories is used to describe the energy released from burning up foodstuffs. There is a conversion factor, though, and calories can be converted into kilojoules if you multiply by 4.2.

Whichever calculation you prefer, the energy stored in each gram of fat is about 9 calories, and every time a gram of fat is burned in your body, 9 calories are released.

When a housewife thinks of fat, she thinks of bacon fat, dripping, lard, or olive oil she uses for frying, or the butter and margarine she buys for the table. However, the housewife's cooking fat is made up of several chemically related but different fatty substances. To avoid the confusion, and to try to be more precise, biochemists and nutritionists invented a new word, lipid, to cover all the related substances a housewife calls fat.

Lipids can be divided into four main groups. These are fatty acids, phospholipids, triglycerides, and sterols. In fact, fatty acids combine with other chemicals to make up the other three lipid compounds. There are more than 40 different fatty acids which are made up of carbon, oxygen, and hydrogen. They occur in the body either as saturated fatty acids or as unsaturated fatty acids. In saturated fatty acids all the carbon atoms are completely saturated with hydrogen atoms. If some of the hydrogen atoms attached to the carbon atoms have been removed, the fatty acid is said to be unsaturated. There is strong evidence that the quantity of saturated fatty acids eaten in the diet is related to the chance of coronary heart disease developing.

Phospholipids are formed from two molecules of fatty acids joined with a molecule of phosphoric acid and held together by a molecule of glycerol (which acts as a kind of glue and is a carbohydrate). Phospholipids help form the walls of the millions of cells which make up the body. They do not appear ever to be in short supply or to cause disease. They also help to disperse lipids into cells and back from cells into the blood plasma.

Triglycerides are made up of three of the fatty acids (as you would expect) and glycerol. Triglycerides are the most usual form of lipids found in plant foodstuffs and in the fat of animals, and consequently they are the usual form of fat you eat. As I mentioned, the fatty acids that make up triglycerides may be mainly saturated or mainly unsaturated, and this can affect your health. Most beef and lamb fat is composed mainly of saturated triglycerides, while fish fat and fowl fat is largely unsaturated.

The most important of the third main group of lipids, the sterols, is a substance called cholesterol. This substance is absent in all foods of plant origin, but is found in all animal foods, and especially in eggs.

Cholesterol is a vital chemical in your body. It is the main ingredient from which you manufacture the bile salts which you need to digest the food you eat. It is the base chemical from which many of the hormones in your body are formed. Only part of the cholesterol is obtained from your diet. Most is synthesized in your body, and this is several times more than the amount you absorb from the food you eat. However, many scientists believe that dietary cholesterol may be dangerous if you eat too much of it. Excess cholesterol, they believe, is in some way connected with heart disease.

As well as making up energy stores in your body, the fat you eat provides the second largest source of the energy you obtain from your diet. People living in Australia, Western Europe, North America, and New Zealand obtain about 40 per cent of their daily needs of calories from fat. An average diet eaten by an active adult provides about 120 g of fat, which will supply you with over 1,000 kilocalories of energy. In the affluent, developed nations about half of this fat is eaten as butter or margarine and about half is 'hidden fat'. Hidden, that is, in cakes, puddings, and pastries. Most Western people find that they need fats in cooking to make their food more palatable. But since fats are relatively expensive, the poorer sections of a society eat less fat than average, and some people eat less than 50 g a day. Since vitamin A is fat-soluble, diets low in fat may be short in vitamin A and vitamin deficiencies may result.

In contrast, most people in the hungry, developing nations eat only small amounts of fat, and the amount rarely exceeds 40 g each day. A diet providing between 40 and 80 g of fat not only provides all the fat needed for good nutrition and supplies all the fat-soluble vitamins you need but avoids the possible dangers of excess fat in the diet. In fact, Western men and women probably eat too much fat. But we enjoy it. Whether we should is another matter.

One of the problems in determining how much or how little fat is really needed is that a diet deficient in fat is also likely to be deficient in protein and other nutrients you need to maintain good health.

Proteins

Proteins make up about 15 per cent of the mass of your body, and are essential for the maintenance and repair of your tissues. The greater the turnover of body tissues, the greater the need is for protein. This means that in infancy and childhood more protein is needed because the body is growing rapidly at that time. If insufficient protein is eaten during the growing period, mental dullness and protein deficiency diseases result. Unfortunately in the developing world very many infants and young children obtain insufficient protein and are malnourished.

Proteins are complex substances made up of simpler substances called amino-acids. There are 23 amino-acids which combine to form proteins. Most proteins contain between 50 and 1,000 molecules of various combinations of amino-acids strung out in a long chain, like a twisted necklace. Every species of plant, and every species of animal, has its characteristic proteins. Plants produce, or more correctly synthesize, all their amino-acids from simple inorganic substances—carbon, nitrogen, oxygen, and hydrogen—but animals are unable to do this, and have to obtain their amino-acids by eating plants or other animals. To a limited extent, animals convert one amino-acid into another in their livers, but there are eight amino-acids which animals cannot make for themselves, and must obtain from their food. Unless these amino-acids are obtained in the diet, protein deficiency diseases may result. These amino-acids are called *essential amino-acids*.

The main source of protein in our Western diet lies in the meat, milk, and eggs we eat. However, animal protein is expensive and the majority of the world's inhabitants get all or nearly all of their protein needs from plants, mainly from cereals and vegetables. Unfortunately most cereal protein lacks one or more of the essential amino-acids, so that to maintain good health, a vegetarian must eat a mixed diet of various cereals, plus nuts and vegetables. If he does this, he will obtain all the essential amino-acids and all the protein he needs, since a lack of an essential amino-acid in one food is made up for by its presence in another food.

The quality of a protein needed for growth during infancy and childhood, and for maintenance of your tissues in adult life, is determined by its amino-acid composition. Animal foods provide all the essential amino-acids in a smaller quantity of food than do cereals, which only contain a small percentage of protein. It has also been found that over 90 per cent of the amino-acids in animal protein are absorbed, but that less than 80 per cent of the amino-acids contained in cereal and vegetable proteins are absorbed. This means that a poor person, who cannot afford to buy meat, eggs, or milk, has to eat a great deal of cereal to obtain the amino-acids he requires to avoid becoming protein deficient. Since the amount of food you eat is largely determined by your energy needs, you may be satiated before you have eaten all the cereal needed to provide the protein. This situation is most likely to arise in children in the developing nations. Adults (except pregnant and lactating women, who have to supply protein to their baby) are rarely affected in this way.

As well as providing the materials your tissues need for growth and repair, the breakdown of protein in your body releases energy: one gram of protein releases about 4.5 calories of energy. The average diet in the developed world provides over 90 g of protein per day, and this is certainly more than is needed to maintain the tissues. The excess is used up to provide extra energy. However, if the diet is deficient of its usual energy source, carbohydrate, as it often is in the developing nations, some of the protein in the diet has to be used for energy and is not available for the repair of the tissues. This means that for health, both protein and carbohydrate (or fat) are generally needed, and it is wasteful to increase the protein intake of a hungry person unless, at the same time, you give him additional carbohydrate.

The effects of energy and protein deficiency (since both usually occur together) can be serious. The deficiencies are more severe in infants after weaning and in young children, although adults, particularly pregnant women, can be affected.

The effects are most marked in tissues which have a rapid turnover of cells, and the gut is one of the tissues most affected, because the cells that make up your gut are formed and destroyed amazingly rapidly.

Protein deficiency upsets the cells lining the gut and damages those cells that produce the enzymes necessary to digest your food. It also reduces a child's resistance to gastro-intestinal infections. The result is that the protein–energy deficient child develops diarrhoea. This makes his condition worse since the limited food he has eaten is less well absorbed as it is hurried through his gut, so the child becomes increasingly deficient in energy and protein. It becomes thin and wasted (or marasmic), or, worse, it may develop kwashiorkor.

Carbohydrates

Carbohydrates are the main source of the energy needed for the human body to function, to power the repair and maintenance of its tissues, to provide the energy needed for activity, and to secure a store of energy which may be needed when food is short. Carbohydrates make up less than 1 per cent of the mass of your body. The amount is small because the carbohydrates provided by food are so rapidly burned up, or are converted into glycerides for storage in fat, or into glycogen for storage in your liver and the glycogen–water pool so that little remains.

In the rich overfed nations, carbohydrates in the diet provide between 50 and 60 per cent of the total calories eaten each day. In the hungry developing nations carbohydrates provide up to 85–90 per cent of the energy needed for one day. In all nations, the poorer you are the more cheap carbohydrates and the less expensive protein (and fat) you eat in your diet. There are few exceptions to this. For example, Eskimos eat very few carbohydrates, because in their environment of snow for most of the year, and tundra for the rest, few are available. They have adapted their diet to meet the environment, and eat large quantities of fat instead. In East Africa the Masai tribe lives on foods of mainly animal origin—eating meat, and drinking milk or blood—and eats very few carbohydrates.

This suggests that carbohydrates are not an essential part of human diets, but for most people they are a favoured form of food. Man, with the exceptions I have mentioned, prefers to eat a mixed diet with proteins, fats, and carbohydrates in varying proportions, depending on cultural, economic, and climatic conditions. It is also certain that most people, in most countries, obtain most of their energy supply by eating carbohydrates.

Carbohydrates are synthesized by plants from water and the

carbon dioxide in the air, under the influence of sunlight. Some of the carbohydrates synthesized are used to make the fibrous tissues—the cellulose or wood, which are the supporting structures of plants. The rest are used for the energy needed for growth, or are stored in the plants in the form of sugar or starch.

Man and other animals are unable to synthesize carbohydrates, but have been remarkably efficient in finding, gathering, and eating edible plants composed mostly of carbohydrates.

About 10,000 years ago man took a giant stride forward in providing himself with a better diet. Somewhere in Asia Minor a man or a woman chose certain seeds of favoured cereals and deliberately planted them. The dawn of agriculture had occurred and it led to an increase in easily available food.

Carbohydrates in foods consist of starches and sugars and fibrous material. The sugars and starches are converted in the body into water and carbon dioxide, releasing energy.

Starch is the most common form of dietary carbohydrate. This is found in all cereal grains and in roots and tubers, such as potatoes and yams. In the human gut, starch is broken down to sugar, ending up as glucose, which is absorbed into your blood. The glucose is either used for immediate energy needs, or it is turned into glycogen. Glycogen is the animal equivalent of the plant storage carbohydrate, starch, and like starch is made up of branching chains of glucose. Glycogen is stored in the liver and in the glycogen–water pool in your muscles. It, rather than fat, is the substance which releases energy should you need it quickly.

Although glucose is the form in which you absorb sugar from the gut, sucrose is the usual form in which sugars are found in plants. Sucrose, the sugar found in sugar-cane and beet, is itself made up of links of one molecule of glucose and one molecule of fruit sugar (fructose).

As I have mentioned, people living in the developing, poorer nations obtain most of their carbohydrates from cereals, tubers, and roots. These foods also contain protein and other nutrients. In the rich overfed world an increasing amount of the carbohydrate eaten comes from surgar-cane or beet. The sucrose obtained is refined so that it is white in colour, and is almost pure carbohydrate. Unlike unrefined cereals, which provide you with protein and other nutrients, pure cane sugar and beet sugar only provide calories, the so-called 'empty calories'.

The sugar addicts, at the moment, form a minority of the world's people. The majority of people eat some sucrose, but get most of their energy from the carbohydrates found in rice, maize, or millet, or in the form of bread, usually made from wheat.

The remnants of the plant wall of cereals, tubers, and most fruits is called fibre. Fibre is composed of celluloses, hemicelluloses, and lignin, and the proportion of each varies in the fibre of different plants.

The fibre content of food can be calculated in two ways. In the first, the fibre is that part of carbohydrate food which is not dissolved by dilute acid or alkali. This is called 'crude fibre'. The second analytical estimate of fibre is more complicated but more accurate. In this method the total 'dietary fibre' is estimated. On average, 'crude fibre' forms about one-quarter of total dietary fibre.

Until recently, nutritionists assumed that fibre was of no importance because it had no energy value, and contained no protein, minerals, or vitamins. It was considered to be merely the material which enabled a plant or a tree to grow erect and to bend with the wind. It was of no importance in the diet of man. At best it added to the bulk of his faeces, at worst it irritated his bowel before being evacuated in his stools.

This belief has been criticized in recent years, particularly since many diseases which afflict affluent people are uncommon in poor nations whose people eat large quantities of unrefined carbohydrate. Unrefined means that the apparently useless fibre has not been removed. In refined carbohydrates such as white flour and white sugar most of the fibre has been removed or is not present.

Scientists began to wonder if the fibre was so useless after all. When refined white flour or white sugar is eaten (which is the normal habit in rich societies, except among health food enthusiasts) the amount of fibre in the cereal or sugar is less than 1 per cent. If wholemeal wheat, or home-ground maize or millet is chosen, the fibre content rises to about 10 per cent. Yet the people who eat the larger amount of 'useless' fibre seem to avoid the many diseases which affect the rich.

Alcoholic drinks

The sugar addicts are not the only addicts who can add substantially to their weight and can damage their health over the
years. The alcohol addicts are an equally important group of
people. From earliest recorded history, and certainly for long
before man made permanent marks on rock, parchment, or
papyrus, he had learnt to use yeast to ferment carbohydrates
and produce a pleasant, stimulating drink containing alcohol in
the form of ethanol (ethyl alcohol). Ethanol is easily metabolized
to release its energy. In moderation it has no long-term harmful
effects. In excess it can be lethal, either directly (by damaging
the liver) or indirectly by causing recklessness and lack of
judgement, for example, when driving a car.

Vitamins

Vitamins have only been discovered in the last 70 years,
although diseases due to deficiency of vitamins have been
described for centuries. Vitamins are organic substances which
the body requires in tiny amounts so that it can continue its
processes of maintenance, repair, and growth. In 1912, when
the first vitamins were discovered, they were thought to be vital
amino-acids (hence the name—*vit-amine*), and each was given a
letter of the alphabet to identify it. That is how vitamin A, which
was found first, was named. Today, the chemical composition
of each vitamin has been established, and each has been given a
chemical name. However, the alphabetical label has stuck, and
most people, including many scientists, continue to refer to
retinol (and carotenoids) as vitamin A; calciferol as vitamin D;
tocopherol as vitamin E; ascorbic acid as vitamin C; thiamine,
riboflavine, niacin, pyridoxine, panthothenic acid, biotin, folic
acid, and cyanocobalamin as various members of the vitamin B
group. In fact, the chemical names of the vitamin B group are
most often read by the general public on the back of breakfast
cereal packages! Vitamins, A, D, and E are soluble in fat. This
means that once you eat them in your diet any excess absorbed
can be stored in the fatty tissues of your body. It also implies that
once you have filled the fat stores you would have to eat a diet
deficient in a fat-soluble vitamin for many months before a
vitamin deficiency disease would arise.

Vitamins B and C are not soluble in fat, but will dissolve in water. Your body cannot keep a large store of water-soluble vitamins, so that if you eat a diet deficient in vitamin C or one of the members of the B group, you are likely to show signs of vitamin deficiency after an interval of weeks rather than months.

Minerals

If all flesh is grass, as the Bible says, the human body also contains certain minerals which are essential for our well-being. The mineral of which we have the greatest amount is calcium. Calcium (together with its constant companion, phosphorus) has to be obtained in your diet so that your bones grow straight during childhood and adolescence and remain strong throughout your life. When you become old your bones may become brittle, and may break. The reasons for this are complex and are discussed in Chapter 5, where you can also find out how you can reduce the chances of this occurring. Your bones (and teeth) contain about 1.2 kg of calcium, mostly in the form of calcium phosphate (which is why I wrote that phosphorus is calcium's constant companion). In fact, nutritionists say, 'if you look after the calcium needs, the requirements for phosphorus look after themselves'. As well as the calcium in bone, a tiny amount of calcium (no more than 10 g) is found in the body fluids and in certain soft tissues, such as the muscles and the nerves of your body. But this tiny quantity of calcium is important, because calcium is essential in the process of blood clotting, in the contraction of muscles, and in the excitability of nerves. Some people, and particularly children with severe rickets, show signs of deficiency of tissue calcium. Their muscles become flabby and they develop spasms in their facial muscles or in those of their hands and feet, a condition known as tetany.

Perhaps the most important mineral in your body as far as health is concerned is iron, yet in your body you have only the amount contained in a large nail. Iron is essential for your survival, mainly because it combines with a protein to form a substance called haemoglobin. Haemoglobin is the pigment in the red blood cells of your body. It carries the oxygen you need from your lungs to the tissues of your body. Iron is also an essential component of a muscle protein called myoglobin, which takes up and releases the oxygen required to make muscles contract. As well as this, minute amounts of iron are important in the enzyme functions of cells.

Other minerals in your body in trace quantities are magnesium, which is also involved in enzyme activity in cells; iodine, which is needed by your body to make the essential thyroid hormones; fluoride, which hardens your teeth and delays dental caries, and zinc, among others.*

Water and electrolytes

Even if all flesh is grass, man is mostly water. Sixty per cent of the weight of your body is water. This means that if you weigh 60 kg, the water in your body will measure 36 litres and weigh 36 kg. Two-thirds of this water is within the millions of cells which make up your body tissues. The remaining third lies outside the cells, making up the fluids of your blood and your lymph, and lying in the narrow spaces between cells. The water in your body is not pure. It contains quantities of sodium, potassium, magnesium, and calcium, usually combined with chloride, which gives it a resemblance to sea water, and perhaps hints at man's maritime origins. When these minerals are dissolved in water they are called electrolytes, and a movement of electrolytes between the water within the cells and that between the cells is constantly happening. The transfer of the electrolytes is essential for the processes which keep the cells alive and functioning, and with each movement of sodium into the cells, or of potassium out of the cells, energy is used.

Salt, in the form of sodium chloride, is the most important electrolyte, and man has either always needed or has been conditioned to eat salt. The singular importance of salt as part of the diet is demonstrated by the fact that for centuries trade in salt was more important than trade in any other commodity. Salt is not only needed to maintain the composition of body water, but is an excellent food preservative. In general, most people eat as much salt as they need to maintain the electrolyte

* The others include copper, cobalt, lead, manganese, molybdenum, selenium, nickel, and arsenic. Deficiency of these minerals is not known to cause any disease in man, although they may poison you if taken in excess.

balance of their body fluids, but habit plays a part. Some primitive groups eat very little salt and seem healthy. In contrast, many Western people eat more salt than they need because custom has habituated the taste buds in their tongue to require salty foods. There is some evidence that an addiction to salt (in temperate climates, at least) may be damaging to health. It has been observed that people living in northern Japan eat twice as much salt as those living in southern Japan. The northern Japanese have a much greater chance of developing high blood pressure and of dying from strokes. This is not to suggest that excessive salt eaten over the years *causes* high blood pressure, but it may be a factor and it does suggest that it would be wise to be abstemious in our use of salt.

The water which makes up the largest proportion of your body comes from the fluid you drink, from the water content of the food you eat, and from the burning up or oxidation of that food in your body. Each gram of starch, when it is used up, releases about 0.6 g of water; each gram of protein utilized releases about 0.4 g of water; and each gram of fat burned up yields just under 1 g of water. Throughout the day you lose fluid from your body. It is lost in the urine you pass, in the sweat which constantly exudes through your skin, in the air you breathe out, and in the fluids you secrete into your gut.

In this way a fluid balance is established: the amount of fluid taken into your body in food and drink, or created by burning up food in your body, is balanced by the amount of fluid you lose. If the balance is upset and you lose more fluid than you obtain, you become dehydrated. In severe cases of dehydration your eyes become sunken, your skin and tongue are dry, your lips are cracked and hard, and your skin loses its elasticity. If you pinch the skin of a dehydrated person it will stand up away from the underlying tissue. Dehydration may occur during fevers, because your body tries to keep your temperature down by increased evaporation of fluid from your skin and your lungs. It occurs in cholera and other diseases causing severe diarrhoea because of the fluid taken from your body by the inflamed cells which line the gut. Dehydration occurs in hot climates if you do not drink enough fluids. In all cases of dehydration, sodium chloride is lost with the water, so you become deficient both in water and in electrolytes.

If the electrolyte and water balance is changed in the opposite direction, you retain more fluid in your body than you lose. When your body water is increased by 10 per cent or more (that is, by about three litres in an average person) the fluid becomes obvious, and a condition called *oedema* results. Your limbs become swollen, especially around the lower legs and ankles and if you press your thumb into the swollen area and keep it pressed for about half a minute, a pit will appear, and will remain for a while after your thumb has been removed.

Energy

It will be obvious that a major function of the diet is to provide energy so that all the cells and organs which compose your body may function properly. The amount of energy required for this varies, depending on your age and your body size, the type of work you do, and the environment in which you work. A 65-year-old woman weighing 50 kg who spends most of her time sitting knitting by the fire requires less energy than a 25-year-old lumberjack who weighs 75 kg and works out of doors in a cold climate. It is perhaps not so obvious that people of the same approximate age and sex, who live in the same environment and have a similar life-style, have similar energy needs whatever their ethnic origin. In England, British-born, West Indian-born, Pakistan-born, Australian-born, and Nigerian-born bus conductors of similar age and body size will have approximately the same energy needs for their work. The main difference in their actual needs is due to the amount of energy they expend during the time—about eight hours—when they are neither in bed nor at work. This non-occupational activity varies considerably from person to person.

Whether you are awake or asleep, whether you are sitting dreaming, or energetically playing a game, you need a constant steady supply of energy for the mechanical work which goes on constantly and unnoticed in your body. Energy is needed for your heart to beat 70 times a minute, 4,200 times an hour, 100,800 times a day, as it forces the oxygen-carrying blood to the tissues and organs of your body. Energy is needed for the muscles of your chest and diaphragm to contract and relax, drawing air in and out of your lungs. Energy is needed for the activities which take place in your gut as food is moved along its nine-metre journey. Energy is needed to maintain the tone of your muscles so that they are ready to contract on demand—for fight or flight! Energy is needed for all the chemical processes that are constantly going on in your body. Energy is needed to keep the cells of your body functioning in an orderly way, so that they can respond immediately and constantly to messages from your brain. Energy is needed to keep your brain functioning, and to maintain your body temperature within very narrow limits.

These energy needs are always present, and energy is expended whether you are active or at rest. In fact, most people spend a large proportion of their day at rest. Rest includes the hours of sleep and the hours when you sit watching the television, reading, or just thinking. The energy expended during this time of rest is that amount needed just to keep the body running. It is called the basal metabolic energy or the basal metabolic rate (BMR). The BMR is defined by physiologists as the energy expended by a person who is relaxed and comfortable soon after waking up in the morning and about 12–14 hours after eating a meal.

Once your basal energy needs have been met, any extra energy you eat (in the form of food) is used for physical activity or is stored as fat. To meet his basal needs, a man requires about 1,700 calories a day, or 1.18 calories a minute. When he undertakes light activity his energy expenditure rises to 2.3 calories a minute, and if he does heavy work the energy he uses goes up to 3.9 calories a minute.

Women need rather less energy for activity because they are usually less heavy and so have a smaller mass to move. For example, women doing housework in the industrialized nations, who have several electrical appliances, are considered to do light activity (many may disagree!) and expend about 1.7 calories a minute. This is the same energy a woman would expend if she worked in an office, was a teacher, or worked in a profession. A woman who has no mechanical household appliances needs more energy for the household jobs she does, and a recent calculation shows that the amount almost exactly equals that she would expend if she worked in light industry.

Most people divide their day into three parts; eight hours

sleep, eight hours work, and eight hours for pottering about, doing 'odd jobs', or watching television. These non-occupational
activities use up energy. Obviously the amount of energy
you use will depend on what you do, so that a range has
to be given.

Your daily energy needs are listed in the following two tables.
These tables are interesting because they show that the difference between the amount of energy expended in doing light
activity and in being very active is only 800 calories. And you
would regain that amount by having three cups of tea each with
three heaped teaspoonfuls of sugar and three ham sandwiches!

If you are a man and weigh less than 65 kg you *deduct* between
40 and 50 calories (depending on your degree of activity) for
every kilogram your weight is below 65 kg to find your energy
requirements. If your weight is more than 65 kg you *add* the
same number of calories for every kilogram your weight exceeds
65 kg.

Energy requirements per day

	Weight in kg	Energy in calories
Children		
less than 1	7.3	820
1–3	13.4	1,360
4–6	20.2	1,830
7–9	28.1	2,190
Male Adolescents		
10–12	36.9	2,600
13–15	51.3	2,900
16–19	62.9	3,070
Female Adolescents		
10–12	38.0	2,350
13–15	49.9	2,490
16–19	54.4	2,310
Adult man moderately active	65.0	3,000
Adult woman moderately active	55.0	2,200
Pregnant woman	Add 285 cals	2,485

Source: W.H.O./F.A.O. *Energy and Protein Requirements* (W.H.O. Tech.
Rep. 522, Rome, 1973), Table 8.

Energy expenditure per day

Activity	Hours	Activity in calories Light (e.g. secretarial or clerical work)	Moderate (e.g. house- work)	Much (e.g. heavy manual labour)
'Reference' man: aged 20–39, weighing 65 kg				
In bed	8	500	500	500
At work	8	1,100	1,400	1,900
Leisure activities	8	1,100	1,100	1,100
Average daily energy expenditure		**2,700**	**3,000**	**3,500**
'Reference' woman: aged 20–39, weighing 55 kg				
In bed	8	420	420	420
At work	8	800	1,000	1,400
Leisure activities	8	780	780	780
Average daily energy expenditure		**2,000**	**2,200**	**2,600**

A similar calculation can be made for women. You must deduct 25 to 40 calories for every kilogram you weigh less than 55 kg; and add 25 to 40 calories for every kilogram you weigh over 55 kg.

As you grow older your body cells become less active, and your resting basal metabolic needs drop slightly. At the same time you are likely to use less energy for non-occupational activities. You sit for longer, and change from playing tennis or squash to golf or bowls, or you become a spectator at sports events rather than being an active participant. This also reduces your daily energy needs with the result that, unless you eat less, you will tend to put on weight.

At the beginning of your life, your energy requirements increase during the period from birth to the age of about 16, when in males the needs reach adult levels. Girls aged 14–18 have an energy requirement about 200–300 calories above that of adult women, because of the great changes occurring in their bodies during puberty and adolescence. If a woman becomes pregnant she also requires extra energy to meet her own needs and those of the foetus, and later her baby if she breast-feeds it.

Glossary

Adipose tissue the tissues of the body which contain large numbers of fat cells. The composition of adipose tissue is 80 per cent fat, 2 per cent protein, and the remainder is water. Because of the high proportion of fat, adipose tissue is often called fatty tissue.

Amino-acids the twenty chemical substances which combine, in an almost infinite number of ways, to produce protein.

Aneurism a weakened, bulging area usually in the wall of the main artery of the body (the aorta).

Appetite the sensation which makes you want to eat a particular food. Often confused with hunger.

Basal metabolic rate (B.M. R.) the energy expended by a person for the vital unconscious processes of the body, which keep it running. These include: heat production, digestion, breathing, and the work of the heart to keep the blood circulating.

Carbohydrates the class of nutrients made up of starches and sugars. See p. 223 for further details.

Defaecate to 'open the bowels' or 'pass a stool'.

Electrolytes see p. 228 for definition.

Energy measurement in kilocalories (as called kcalories, kcals, or calories). A kcal is the amount of heat required to raise the temperature of a litre of water from 15°C. to 16°C.

Enzymes chemical substances produced in the body which are essential to cause chemical transformation of material in plants and animals.

F.A.O. the Food and Agricultural Organization (of the United Nations).

Fetus the growing baby while still in its mother's uterus.

Fibre that part of the plant which is not digested by man. This includes the plant cell wall (lignin) and parts of the cell (some polysaccharides).

Glycogen the form in which excess carbohydrate is stored in the body.

Gram a measure of weight, equivalent to $\frac{1}{28}$th of an ounce. Usually abbreviated to g.

Hunger the sensation which makes you want to eat. Often confused with appetite.

Incidence the number of 'cases' in a given community occurring (or being detected) in a specific period, usually one year.

Lactation the production, secretion, and discharge of milk from the breast.

Lipids the biochemical term for fats (see p. 217 for full discussion).

Nutrition the action or process of receiving substances which promote tissue growth and repair, thus promoting the well-being of the body.

Oedema the swelling of tissues owing to fluid lying in the spaces between the cells which make up the tissue.

Parboiled the rice (still in the husk) is steamed before it is milled. This 'fixes' thiamine to the grain and milling does not remove it.

Polyunsaturated fatty acids see p. 219.

Prevalence the number of 'cases' in a given community, usually expressed as the number of every 1,000 population.

Primates animals, closest to man in the evolutionary scale, i.e. apes and monkeys.

Protein see p. 221 for definition.

Saturated fatty acids see p. 219.

Triglycerides a substance made up of three (tri) fatty acids linked and held by glycerol (monoglycerides have only *one* fatty acid linked with glycerol).

W.H.O. the World Health Organization (of the United Nations).

References

1 Fat people are fat because . . .
The complex factors involved in the development of obesity are discussed in detail in *Energy Balance and Obesity in Man* (Elsevier, London, 1975) by J. S. Garrow, and in *Obesity* (Churchill Livingstone, Edinburgh, 1974), edited by W. L. Burland, P. D. Samuel, and J. Yudkin. The quotations by G. V. Mann appear in the *American Journal of Public Health* (61, 1491, 1972). The concept of the glycogen-water pool is discussed by J. S. Garrow (op. cit.), and the relationship between obesity and inactivity by B. A. Bullen in the *American Journal of Clinical Nutrition* (14, 211, 1964).

Childhood obesity and its possible genetic origins is discussed by A. G. C. Whitelaw in the *British Medical Journal* (1, 985, 1976), and by S. M. Garth and D. C. Clark in *Pediatrics* (57, 443, 1976). The relationship between childhood obesity and adult obesity is controversial. It is discussed by C. G. D. Brook in the *British Medical Journal* (2, 25, 1972); in the *Lancet* (2, 1352, 1977); by E. M. Poskitt and T. J. Cole in the *British Medical Journal* (1, 7, 1977); by J. L. Kittle in the *American Journal of Clinical Nutrition* (30, 762, 1977); and, earlier, by J. Hirsch in *Lipid Research* (10, 77, 1969). The emotional factors which may be involved in obesity receive attention from S. Schachter in *Science* (161, 517, 1970). The observation that diet fails to reduce weight in some people received attention from D. S. Miller and S. Parsonage in the *Lancet* (1, 773, 1975). The exercise equivalent of foods is given in a book by F. Koniski with that title published by Southern Illinois University Press, Carbondale, in 1973. Exercise as a means of treating obesity is considered by G. Gwinup in the *Archives of Internal Medicine* (135, 676, 1975). The mistakes made by mothers in feeding their infants have been noted by L. S. Taitz in the *Lancet* (2, 712, 1977), and reconsidered by M. De Swiet in the *Lancet* (1, 892, 1977), and by R. A. K. Jones and E. M. Belsey in the *British Medical Journal* (2, 112, 1976).

2 Breast is best
The biochemical composition of human and cow's milk is described in detail by S. J. Foman in *Infant Nutrition* (Saunders, Philadelphia, 1967), and more recently by D. B. and E. F. P. Jelliffe in *Human Milk in the Modern World* (Oxford University Press, Oxford, 1978). The quotation at the beginning of the chapter is also from the Jelliffes in the *American Journal of Clinical Nutrition* (24, 1018, 1971). Nursing songs are mentioned by N. Newton in the *American Journal of Clinical Nutrition*

(24,993,1971). The dangers of faulty preparation of cow's 'formula milk' has received a good deal of attention, most recently in *Present Day Practices in Infant Feeding*, a report by the Department of Health and Social Security (H.M.S.O., London, 1975), and by R. K. Oates in the *British Medical Journal* (2, 642, 1973). The survey made in 1970 by J. A. G. Anderson and A. Gatherer and reported in the *British Medical Journal* (2, 20, 1970) has been followed by others which have shown the same pattern, e.g. R. A. K. Jones and E. M. Belsey, in the *British Medical Journal* (2, 112, 1976).

The protective effect of human milk against gastro-intestinal and respiratory infections in infants is well established. It is discussed by D. B. and E. F. B. Jelliffe (op. cit.); by J. D. Wray in *Paediatrics* (55, 723, 1975); by L. Hambraeus in *Acta Paediatrica Scandinavica* (67, 561, 1978); and by J. F. Robinson in the *British Medical Journal* (1, 1443, 1978). The value of breast-feeding as a method of birth control is noted in *The Nutrition Factors*, by A. Berg (Brookings Institute, Washington, 1973), and by F. W. Rosa in an article in the *P. A. G. Bulletin* (F. A. O., Rome, July 1975).

The decline in breast-feeding is widely documented: in the U.S.A. by H. P. Meyer in *Clinical Paediatrics* (7, 708, 1968); in Britain by E. Eastham in the *British Medical Journal* (1, 305, 1976); in Sweden by P. O. Peterson and G. von Sydow in the *British Medical Journal* (3, 490, 1975); and in Australia by D. B. Newton in the *Medical Journal of Australia* (1, 801, 1966). The prevalence of breast-feeding in primitive races is recorded by C. S. Ford in his book *A Comparative Study of Human Reproduction* (Hale University Press, New Haven, 1945) and in the *P. A. G. Bulletin*, No. 3 (F.A.O., Rome, 1973).

The modest return to breast-feeding is documented in the Annual Reports of the Victorian Department of Health, Australia.

More details of the physiology of lactation may be found in R. M. Applebaum's article in *Paediatric Clinic of North America* (17, 203, 1970). Infant feeding practices occurring in hospitals are documented by Doris and John Haire in *The Nurse's Contribution to Breast-Feeding* (International Childbirth Education Foundation, New Jersey, 1974) and by P. De Chateau in *Developmental Medicine and Child Neurology* (19, 575, 1977). The attitudes of mothers towards breast-feeding are documented by N. and M. Newton in *Paediatrics* (5, 869, 1960); by E. J. Salber and J. Feinlieb in *Journal of Paediatrics* (37, 299, 1976); and by L. J. Newson and E. Newson in the *British Medical Journal* (2, 1974, 1962).

Recent recognition of the importance of early bonding between mother and baby and its effect on subsequent development is described in *Maternal-Infant Bonding* by M. H. Klaus and J. H. Kennell (C. V. Mosby, Saint Louis, 1976).

The help and support provided for home-based nursing mothers by voluntary community organizations cannot be underestimated. The

Nursing Mothers' Association of Australia, the La Leche League International in the U.S.A., and the National Childbirth Trust in the U.K. offer counselling and advice to mothers who have problems when breast-feeding. In many cities a telephone counsellor is 'on call' twenty-four hours a day. The La Leche League has its head office in Chicago; the National Childbirth Trust has its head office in London; and the Nursing Mothers' Association of Australia has its head office in Melbourne.

3   Our daily bread
The source book of the history of bread is *White Bread and Brown* by R. A. McCance and E. M. Widdowson (Pitman Medical, London, 1956). The cultivation of cereals, beginning in three centres in the world, is noted by J. R. Harlen in *Science* (174, 468, 1971); while T. McKeown describes the changes in agriculture after 1700 in *Demography* (26, 345, 1972), and in *Population Studies* (32, 535, 1978). The Wuppertal 'experiment' was reported by R. A. McCance and E. M. Widdowson in *Studies of Under-nutrition* (Medical Research Council, Special Report No. 275, 1951 and No. 287, 1954).

The effects of bran on human health has received considerable attention since 1970, notably by D. P. Burkett in, for example, the *British Medical Journal* (1, 274, 1973) and in the *Lancet* (2, 1408, 1972). Dr Payler reported beneficial effects of bran in the *Lancet* (1, 1394, 1973), but the 'bran hypothesis' was criticized by M. A. Eastwood in the *Lancet* (1, 1029, 1974), and by P. Soltoff in the *Lancet* (1, 920, 1976). The hypothesis was supported by R. F. Harvey in the *Lancet* (1, 1278, 1973), and by A. R. P. Walker in the *Postgraduate Medical Journal* (49, 242, 1973). The controversy about the relationship of the diet to bowel cancer is discussed in the *Lancet* (2, 208, 1977), and by E. L. Wynder in *Cancer* (3, 80, 1974). The effect of diet on the incidence of varicose veins is discussed in *On the Causation of Varicose Veins* by T. L. Cleave (Wright, Bristol, 1960), and by C. Latto in the *Lancet* (1, 1089, 1973).

A careful well-written study of the health implications of the fibre in our diet is found in *Refined Carbohydrate Foods and Disease—Some Implications of Dietary Fibre* (Academic Press, London, 1975) by D. P. Burkitt and H. C. Trowell.

4   A sweet but deadly addiction
The possible consequences to health of a diet which contains a considerable amount of sugar is discussed in *Pure, White and Deadly* (Davis-Poynter, London, 1973) by John Yudkin, who has also edited *Sugar: Chemical, Biological and Nutritional Aspects of Sucrose* (Butterworth, London, 1971). The high prevalence of dental decay amongst children in the U.K., the U.S.A., and Australia is noted by A. Sheilham (*British Dental Journal*, 9, 401, 1969); by the *National Centre for Health Statistics* (Ser. 11, No. 7, Washington, 1965); and by P. D. Barnard (*Australian Dental Journal*, 1, 274, 1974). The effect on dental caries of reducing

sugar in the diet has been discussed by many authors, notably R. L. Hartles and S. A. Leach (*British Medical Bulletin*, 31, 137, 1975) and A. J. W. McKendrick (*Lancet*, 2, 1087, 1975).

Diabetes continues to be a matter of health concern. Its prevalence in the community seems to be increasing, according to R. R. Rodriques and J. Vallence-Owen in *Diabetes* (Excerpta Medica, Amsterdam, 1971); M. E. Wadsworth (*Lancet*, 2, 1172, 1974); and H. Trowell (*Lancet*, 2, 998, 1974 and 2, 1510, 1974). The problem is also discussed by T. L. Cleeve and G. D. Campbell in *Diabetes, Coronary Thrombosis and the Saccharine Disease* (Wright, Bristol, 1969). The reason why a sugar-rich diet should provoke diabetes is discussed by A. B. Wicks and J. J. Jones (*British Medical Journal*, 1, 773, 1973).

5 Two valuable minerals
The effect of the loss of calcium from bones as people age (especially women) is discussed by H. C. Gallagher and B. E. C. Nordin in *Ageing and Oestrogens* (Karger, Basle, 1973). The problem of prescribing oestrogen to reduce bone loss is controversial. J. M. Atkins (*British Medical Journal*, 3, 515, 1973) believes that the protection offered by oestrogen outweighs the risk of developing uterine cancer. The relationship between oestrogen and uterine cancer was noted by H. K. Zeil and W. D. Finkle (*American Journal of Obstetrics and Gynaecology*, 124, 735, 1976).

Anaemia is a common disease and, usually, is due to a lack of iron in the diet, or to a loss of iron from haemorrhage. A good discussion is found in *Nutritional Anaemias* (W.H.O. Tech. Rep. Ser. 405, 1968; 452, 1970; 503, 1972). The prevalence of anaemia in the community is shown by L. Hallberg in *Iron Deficiency Anaemias* (Academic Press, London, 1970), and *Occurrence, Causes and Prevention of Nutritional Anaemias* (Alinquist and Wiksell, Stockholm, 1968).

The original research by Lucy Wills in India was reported in the *British Medical Journal* (1, 1059, 1931).

6 An A, D, E, B, C of vitamins
A general discussion of vitamin deficiency is found in A. W. Franklin's chapter in *The History and Conquest of Common Diseases*, edited by W. E. Bett (University of Oklahoma Press, 1954), and in P. Greengard's chapter in *The Pharmacological Basis of Therapeutics*, edited by L. S. Goodman and A. Gilman (Macmillan, New York, 1970).

Rickets is considered in detail by A. E. Hess in his book *Rickets* (Lea and Seberger, Philadelphia, 1929), and in an article by E. Kodicek (*Lancet*, 1, 325, 1974).

The need for vitamin E is evaluated by J. Howitt in *Vitamins and Hormones* (20, 541, 1962; 26, 487, 1968); and by both the National Academy of Sciences in the U.S.A. and the Food and Nutrition Board, Division of Biology and Agriculture (National Research Council, June 1973).

The history of the discovery of thiamine deficiency as the cause of beri-beri appears in an article by R. E. Byron in *Studies from the Institute for Medical Research, Federation of Malaya* (25, 98, 1951). D. Roe writes about pellagra in *A Plague of Corn* (Cornell University Press, New York, 1973).

The story of scurvy in the Royal Navy is based largely on the writings of C. Lloyd and J. L. S. Coulter in volume 3 of *Medicine and the Navy* (E. and S. Livingstone, Edinburgh, 1961). Linus Pauling has written extensively about man's need for large amounts of vitamin C: his views are summarized in *Vitamin C, the Common Cold and the 'Flu* (W. H. Freeman, San Francisco, 1977).

The effectiveness of vitamin C in reducing the incidence of the common cold was evaluated in an editorial in the *British Medical Journal* (1, 606, 1976).

If large doses of vitamin C do reduce the discomfort of a cold, which seems unlikely, scientists can only speculate how it works. For example, C. W. H. Wilson (*Lancet*, 2, 859, 1973) thinks that vitamin C may improve the efficiency of the phagocytes—the cells which scavenge and eliminate bacteria from the blood, or that it may increase a person's immunity to viruses in an undiscovered way. M. Briggs (*Lancet*, 2, 677, 1973) points out that ascorbic acid dissolves easily and quickly in water, and so passes very easily into body fluids, including mucus. He thinks that the vitamin may soften mucus in the lung tubes, and this could be a reason why some people taking vitamin C have less severe colds and feel better at the height of a cold.

7   An insufficiency of energy, a paucity of protein
The effects of protein-energy malnutrition are discussed in the P.A.G. Bulletins (F.A.O., Rome, 1972 onwards); in A. Berg's book *The Nutrition Factor* (Brookings Institute, Washington D.C., 1973); in *Lives in Peril: Protein and the Child* (F.A.O., Rome, 1970); in *Patterns of Mortality in Childhood* by R. R. Putter and C. V. Serrano (P.A.H.O. (W.H.O.) Scientific Publication, Washington, 262, 1973). The prevalence of malnutrition has been reported and discussed in many publications. A good example is an article in *Science* (181, 634, 1973).

The protein requirements of individuals is discussed by A. E. Bender (*Lancet*, 2, 595, 1974). The possible damaging effect of maternal and infant protein malnutrition on the intellectual capacity of infants receive attention from J. Dobbing (*Lancet*, 1, 803, 1974), M. B. Stoch and P. H. Smythe (*Archives of Diseases of Childhood*, 51, 327, 1976), and J. Hoorweg and J. P. Stanfield (*Developmental Medicine and Child Neurology*, 13, 330, 1976). A balanced assessment of this complex problem can be found in *Early Malnutrition and Mental Development*, a symposium of the Swedish Nutrition Foundation (vol. 12, 1974).

Marasmus and kwashiorkor are differentiated by J. C. Waterlow in a letter to the *Lancet* (2, 712, 1974) and by J. F. Brock (*Lancet*, 2, 713, 1974).

8 The fats of death?

The different prevalence of coronary heart disease in various nations is examined by J. Stammler in *Ischaemic Heart Disease* (ed. J. H. Hass, Leiden University Press, 1970), and by R. A. B. Drury (*Tropical Geographical Medicine*, 24, 382, 1972). The increased amount of fat and sucrose in the diet during the past century are noted by M. A. Antar and D. F. Hollingsworth (*American Journal of Clinical Nutrition*, 14, 169, 1964; 20, 65, 1967). How atherosclerosis begins remains speculative. Theories are discussed by Dr J. I. Mann, Sir John McMichael, and Sir George Pickering in the *British Medical Journal* (1, 732, 1979; 1, 180, 1979; 1, 1025, 1979). The pathological changes in the arteries, leading to atherosclerosis, are reviewed by R. Russell and J. A. Glomset in *Science* (180, 1332, 1973), by J. C. Lewis and B. A. Kottke in *Science* (196, 1007, 1979), and by R. Ross and J. A. Glomset in *New England Journal of Medicine* (295, 420, 1977).

The case against animal saturated fats as a major factor in coronary heart disease received wide support, notably from the Intersociety Commission for Heart Disease Resources in the U.S.A. which published its findings in *Circulation* (42, A-55, 1970). W. B. Kannel, who has been associated with the Framingham study since its inception, recorded his views in *Annals of Internal Medicine* (74, 1971), and later in the *Journal of the American Medical Association* (227, 338, 1974). The protective effect of high-density lipids was described by N. E. Miller (*Lancet*, 1, 965, 1977) and in an editorial in the *Lancet* (2, 1291, 1978).

The main protagonist arguing that sucrose is a major risk factor in coronary heart disease, J. Yudkin, has published many papers. His views are summarized in his book *Pure, White and Deadly* (Davis-Poynter, London, 1973). G. D. Campbell also writes with conviction about this relationship in *Diabetes, Coronary Thrombosis and the Saccharine Disease* (Wright, Bristol, 1966).

The risk factors in coronary heart disease are discussed in great detail in several publications, which also have large bibliographies. In Britain, two reports are available: 'Prevention of Coronary Heart Disease' (*Journal of the Royal College of Physicians*, 10, 213, 1976) and *Diet and Coronary Heart Disease* (Department of Health and Social Security, H.M.S.O., 1974). The former was compiled by a joint working party of the Royal College of Physicians and the Cardiac Society.

9 Crazy diets and dietary crazes

The American magazine *Consumer's Guide* has published an excellent analysis of no fewer than sixty-two diets, mainly available in book form. *Rating the Diets*, by Theodore Berland (Publications International Limited, Skokie, Ill., 1975) gives details of most of the diets discussed in this chapter.

10 A sensible diet for Mr, Ms, Mrs

Weight Watchers International has branches in many cities in most developed nations, as has TOPS. While they achieve considerable success with their regimens, some people still fail to lose weight, as recorded by D. S. Miller and S. Parsonage (*Lancet*, 1, 773, 1975) and H. Curry (*Journal of the American Medical Association*, 237, 2829, 1977). Some of these people may be helped by behavioural modification. This is discussed by R. B. Stuart and B. Davis in *Slim Chance in a Fat World* (Research Press, Champaign, Ill., 1971). The place of drugs in controlling obesity is considered by D. Craddock in *Current Therapeutics* (71, 87, Feb. 1976). The hormone HCG is advocated persuasively by A. T. W. Simeons in the *Lancet* (2, 946, 1971), as well as in many other writings. His views have been criticized by J. C. Ballin and P. L. White (*Journal of the American Medical Association*, 4 Nov. 1974) and by E. Drenick, speaking at a symposium of the American Society of Bariatric Physicians in Las Vegas in 1974. Surgery to treat obesity is currently controversial, and was discussed at a symposium in 1977, reported in the *American Journal of Nutrition* (30, 1–130, 1977). It was also discussed at a meeting of the Arthritis Foundation, reported in the *Journal of the American Medical Association* (240, 98, 1978). Anybody contemplating starting on a diet would benefit by reading J. Yudkin's helpful book *This Slimming Business* (Penguin, London, 1971).

Appendix   The food we eat

Human Nutrition and Dietetics by S. Davidson, R. Passmore, and J. F. Brock (5th edn., Churchill Livingstone, Edinburgh, 1973) is the standard English text on human nutrition. It is written in an easily readable style, with delightful anecdotes, but is designed for people who have some knowledge of biochemistry and dietetics. *Energy and Protein Requirements* (W.H.O. Tech. Rep. 522. F.A.O. Nutrition Meeting Rep. 52. Rome, 1973) is the latest in a series of discussions by world experts. *Nutrition for Developing Countries*, edited by Maurice King (Oxford University Press, London, 1972) is a text on the elements of nutrition designed for high school students, nurses, and interested people living in the developing nations. However, it is a useful primer for those interested in human nutrition, and presupposes no scientific knowledge. Alas, it lacks an index! *Nutrition and Its Disorders* by D. S. McLaren (Churchill Livingstone, Edinburgh, 1972) is a short handbook on nutrition which demands a certain amount of biochemical and medical knowledge in the reader.

Index

Adipose cells, 13, 217, 235
Adipose tissue, 5, 217, 218
Alcohol, 211, 226
Amino-acids, 221, 235
Anaemia
    effect on pregnancy, 92, 96
    folic acid and, 100
    incidence in community, 95
    iron deficiency, 93–8
    liver treatment of, 100
    megaloblastic, 99–101
    nutritional, 94
    pernicious, 101
    vitamin C and, 99
Analgesics, 92
Aneurism, 235
'Artificial milks', see Formula milks
Appendicitis, 52, 54
Ascorbic acid, see Vitamin C
Atherosclerosis, 149–52

Basal metabolic rate (BMR), 12, 231, 235
Beri-beri, 119–21
    symptoms, 119
    vitamin B_1 in, 121
Biliharziasis, 98
Blindness, vitamin deficiency, 107
Bone
    calcium and, 85–9
    decalcification of, 88
Bowel
    cancer, 53, 56
    irritated, 55
Brain growth and malnutrition, 142–3
Bran, 53, 56; see also Fibre
Bread
    Assize of, 46
    brown, 46–7
    fortification of, 61, 97, 123
    history, 45–7, 50
    nutritional value, 48
    white, 46, 49
    wholemeal, 48, 60

Wuppertal experiment, 47
Breakfast cereals, 175
Breast-feeding
    attitudes to, 30, 35, 38
    benefits, 23–9
    bonding and, 36
    breast shape and, 30
    contraceptive effect of, 27
    decline in, 29, 35; reasons for, 30, 31, 38
    in developed nations, 29
    duration of, 39, 68
    education for, 41–2
    encouragement of, 36–8, 41
    fertility and, 28
    hospital practices and, 35, 37–8
    prudishness and, 30, 31
    reasons for, 22–9
Breast milk
    allergies and, 24
    anti-infective properties, 25–7
    biochemical composition, 42
    uniqueness of, 22–4
    see also Lactation
Breasts
    anatomy, 32
    engorgement, 38
    erotic nature of, 21, 30
    shape, 30

Calcium, 85–90, 227
    in bone, 89
    in diet, 89
    foods containing, 90
    metabolism of, 86
Carbohydrates
    biochemistry, 223–4
    'refined', 53, 59, 66, 77–8, 155, 191
Calories, 6, 7, 16, 218
    'empty', 65, 172, 175, 211, 224
Cholesterol, 156–60, 173, 220
Cigarette smoking, 165–6, 180
Coca Cola, 80
Cod-liver oil, 109

Acknowledgements

Cartoons by Beny Kandler.

*Drawings on pp. 34 and 35 reprinted by permission of
Faber & Faber Ltd., from* Everywoman by Derk Llewellyn-Jones,
illustrated by Audrey Besterman.